What to Do If You
Get Breast Cancer

What to Do If You Get Breast Cancer

Lydia Komarnicky, M.D., and Anne Rosenberg, M.D., with Marian Betancourt

Little, Brown and Company
Boston • *New York* • *Toronto* • *London*

Acknowledgments

I would like to thank my parents and my husband, Bill, for giving me encouragement and support. I also want to thank Dr. Carl Mansfield for enhancing my career. His expertise and training have proven invaluable. — L.K.

I want to thank my family, parents, and my few true friends for their patience, moral support, and confidence. It's been a long road. — A.R.

Thanks to the women who shared their stories, to Amy Fastenberg for her belief in this book, and to Barbara DeLuca, Marc Rudoltz, M.D., Kathy Schwarz, and Linda Miller for their help. — M.B.

First Edition

The authors are grateful for permission to include the following previously copyrighted material:

Excerpts from *Recovery in Motion* by Linda T. Miller, PT. Copyright © by Linda T. Miller, PT. By permission of the author.

Library of Congress Cataloging-in-Publication Data

Komarnicky, Lydia.
    What to do if you get breast cancer / Lydia Komarnicky and Anne Rosenberg
    with Marian Betancourt. — 1st ed.
      p. cm.
    Includes bibliographical references.
    ISBN 0-316-09288-6 (hc)
    ISBN 0-316-09289-4 (pb)
    1. Breast — Cancer — Popular works. I. Rosenberg, Anne.
    II. Betancourt, Marian. III. Title.
    RC280.B8K37 1995
    616.99'449 — dc20   94-15964

10 9 8 7 6 5 4 3 2 1

MV-NY

Published simultaneously in Canada by Little, Brown & Company (Canada) Limited

Printed in the United States of America

To my son, Alex, and my daughter, Kristen, it is my hope that continued research will permit Kristen to grow up in a society where breast cancer can be prevented. And to all my wonderful patients who have entrusted me with their care. — L.K.

To my sons, Ryan and Evan, who make my life so special, and to the patients, now friends, who have given me their trust and taught me the meaning of life. — A.R.

To my granddaughters, Hilary and Julia, my daughter, Karen, my son, Thomas, and to the women in my breast cancer support groups. — M.B.

Contents

III   Recovery: What to Expect After Treatment

~

Introduction

It wasn't very long ago that a woman might go into the hospital for a breast biopsy and come out without her breast. This cannot happen today. It is now illegal for a doctor or hospital to perform surgery without the patient's written permission and informed consent. Furthermore, amputation of the breast is no longer the only way to deal with breast cancer. Attitudes and techniques have changed, and today women with breast cancer have many more options and much more control than in the past. When little was known and less was written about breast cancer, a woman rarely even knew what to ask about treatment. Breast cancer was not something she talked about. She had her mastectomy and hoped for the best. Her feelings and fears were never discussed.

We — that is, Lydia Komarnicky, a radiation oncologist, and Anne Rosenberg, a breast surgeon — began to devote ourselves to the treatment of breast cancer because we saw too many physicians fail to understand the difference between breast cancer and all other cancer. Few were sensitive to the intricacies of the disease or the dynamics of its effect. Few took the time to talk with patients, to listen or care. There was little awareness of the importance of communicating, of patient and physician working together as a team.

In medical school and residency training in the late 1970s, treating all types of patients, we were drawn to breast cancer patients and became involved in clinical research. Even then, just fifteen years ago, breast cancer was still in the closet. Afflicted women were isolated and frightened and poorly informed. We found ourselves spending more time with these women, listening, talking, helping to explain options. We felt we were on the right path.

Breast cancer is one of the few cancers where doctors *can* make a difference, especially when it is caught early. It is one of the more curable cancers when doctor and patient are well informed. As women we feel a special bond with our patients and their families. We try to give them not only the treatment they need, but also the emotional support that is so important. Every day we are inspired by our patients, by women who ask questions, fight back, refuse to settle. Women who take charge.

The writer of this team, Marian Betancourt, is one of these women. Until breast cancer happened to her, she knew little about it. She soon realized that most women knew even less than she did. As a professional writer, she knew she had a mission. Her energy and talent made this book possible because she wanted others to know "what to do if you get breast cancer."

The diagnosis of breast cancer is shocking enough, but when you are overwhelmed with questions — Will I survive? How do I make the right decision? — you may panic. We hope this book is a place to start, to get information. It is meant to be a practical guide, straightforward and accessible, for women of all ages and backgrounds who have been diagnosed with cancer. We want to walk you through the process from discovery to recovery so that you know what to expect. You need to know exactly what kind of breast cancer you have (there are many), how your pathology report can help you make decisions, and what radiation therapy and chemotherapy are like and when and how they are used. You need to know the surgical options from treatment to reconstruction, what to do if you are pregnant, and how breast cancer affects the rest of your life. We hope this book will help you ask the right questions and help you participate in the decision-making process about your own disease. As an informed patient, you can feel more comfortable with your doctors' recommendations and your own choices for treatment. You can take charge.

Every year nearly 200,000 women in the United States get breast cancer. The majority of us survive, and the number of survivors grows every year. Remember that!

~

Authors' Note

This book is meant to inform and educate; it is not meant to be an alternative to appropriate medical care. The authors have made every effort to insure that the information presented is accurate and up-to-date. But keep in mind that new research findings and information may revise some of this information.

∼ 1

Discovery:
First Find Out What Kind of
Breast Cancer You Have

~ 1

Where to Go If You Find a Lump in Your Breast

Finding a lump in the breast is the way most women discover breast cancer. Although most lumps turn out to be benign (noncancerous), many are not. When diagnosed with breast cancer, most women panic. They want it out — now! You *do* have time to get more information, talk to others who have been treated, consider your options, and make the best choices you can. Breast cancer is treatable and, if detected early enough, curable. Treatment is improving all the time, and survival rates increase every year. Some treatments are controversial, so take the time to find the best treatment available for your particular condition. You will know what is right for you if you learn all you can about what's available and trust your instincts.

A lump in your breast is not the only sign of breast cancer. Any change in your breast needs investigation:

- a lump *near* your breast, including your underarm, collarbone, and neck
- a change in the size or shape of your breast
- redness or swelling of your breast
- discharge from your nipple

3

- puckered or dimpled skin
- ulcerated or inverted nipple or areola
- a thickening or density in your breast or underarm

Start with your family doctor or the doctor with whom you feel most comfortable. If you have no primary physician or gynecologist, call a women's health network or medical center in your area and ask for doctors with *experience in treating breast disease*. There must be one physician who can examine your breast and get you started with the appropriate tests. Ask this doctor for referrals to help you set up the necessary appointments.

Your doctor will usually order a mammogram, an X ray of the breast. But a mammogram may not always show the lump that you can feel. For instance, if a lump is near the lower crease of your breast, it might be missed if not enough of your breast is pulled into the range of the X ray. In that case, a view from another angle is needed. An ultrasound examination is often done to distinguish between a cyst (which is fluid-filled) and a solid tumor. You're not off the hook until the cause of the lump is absolutely explained. Then you can find out treatment options. Most abnormalities will require evaluation by a surgeon, and generally a surgical biopsy. This is outpatient surgery that allows the surgeon to remove a piece of the tumor so a pathologist can test it for cancer. There are general surgeons as well as surgeons who specialize in diseases of the breast. You are most likely to find surgeons experienced with breast cancer in comprehensive cancer centers, large medical centers, big cities, and teaching hospitals.

Your course of action begins with a series of examinations and tests called a workup. This is to identify your cancer and stage it (that is, learn whether it has spread), and can include a mammogram, biopsy, chest and other X rays, as well as several blood tests. These, then, are the steps you might expect to take over the weeks following detection of a lump or other abnormality in your breast:

- Arrange for a physical exam with your primary doctor.
- Get a mammogram (and possibly an ultrasound).
- Talk with your primary doctor again to discuss the findings.
- Visit a breast surgeon for examination.
- Get a biopsy, then a workup.
- Discuss findings and treatment options with a surgeon.
- Join a breast cancer support group.
- Visit other surgeons for second and third opinions.
- Meet and talk with the physicians who will administer radiation (radiation oncologist), chemotherapy (medical oncologist), and possibly plastic surgery.
- Rearrange your work and home schedules.
- Begin treatment.

These organizations can provide referrals to physicians and facilities in your area with experience in breast cancer:

- **American Cancer Society**   800-ACS-2345
Ask for the telephone number of your local chapter.
- **NABCO Hotline**   212-719-0154
National Alliance of Breast Cancer Organizations, based in New York; a veritable encyclopedia of information and referrals on breast cancer.
- **NCI Cancer Information
Service Hotline**   800-4-CANCER
The National Cancer Institute's information and referral network.
- **Y-ME National Hotline**   800-221-2141
Chicago-based referral and support network with several regional hotlines. See Appendix 4 for regional Y-ME numbers.

The First Step After Diagnosis Is Information

Buy a notebook so you can keep track of everything you will need to know. You will be bombarded with information — and sometimes misinformation. Before you can choose the best treatment, you need to know what kind of breast cancer you have. There are several kinds, from small tumors involving a few of the breast ducts or lobules to inflammatory cancer involving the entire breast. Many variables guide treatment planning: size, type, and location of tumor; cell behavior; lymph node involvement; possible metastasis (spreading). "Staging" is the sum of these variables and a determination of any evidence that the breast cancer has spread elsewhere. Your treatment will depend on the dynamics of your breast cancer, as well as your age, general health, temperament, and lifestyle.

Several physicians may be involved in your treatment: surgical oncologist, radiation oncologist, medical oncologist, possibly a plastic reconstructive surgeon. The pathologist plays a role behind the scenes. These physicians all lend their expertise and opinions along the way. This is your treatment team, along with an assortment of technicians, nurses, and other healthcare professionals. Keep in mind, this is your team and you are the captain. Your treatment will be planned in two ways — local treatment and systemic treatment. Local treatment focuses on the actual cancer in your breast and can include surgery (lumpectomy, lymph node dissection, mastectomy) and radiation. Systemic treatment focuses on the rest of your body and is planned if you have a cancer that *can* or has spread to other organs. This is chemotherapy (cytotoxic drugs, hormonal drugs, bone marrow transplant).

Understanding the Anatomy of Your Breast

Your breast has fifteen to twenty lobes, or sections, radiating out from your nipple like the sections of an orange. Each lobe has many smaller divisions, called lobules, which end in dozens of tiny milk-producing bulbs. The lobes, lobules, and bulbs are all linked by thin tubes called ducts, which lead to the nipple. Blood vessels, lymphatics, and nerves run through the breast tissue. The rest of your breast is mostly fatty tissue. Muscles cover your ribs and lie under your breast, but they are not part of your breast.

About 85 percent of cancers arise from the ducts of the breast and are called *ductal carcinoma*. The left breast seems to be a little more vulnerable to breast cancer than the right one and the upper outer quadrant of the breast is where 50 percent of cancers appear. Ten percent appear in each of the other three quadrants, and about 20 percent are in the center of the breast or beneath the areola. Most tumors take years to develop, but some — about 20 percent — are fast growing and can double in size in weeks.

You will be learning a new language now, and it's a good idea to know some of the basic terminology. We'll explain more as we go. The cancerous lump is usually called a carcinoma. Some rare and unusual lumps have other names, like sarcoma. The *primary* is the original site of the cancer. If there are other lumps or lesions involved, then your breast cancer may be *multifocal* or *multicentric*. *Multifocal* means there are additional cancer lesions or cells near the primary, in the same quadrant. *Multicentric* means there are additional lesions or cells in another quadrant of your breast. (A lesion is a tumor, mass, or other abnormality.)

For the purposes of diagnosis, your breast is divided into four sections, or quadrants: upper outer, upper inner, lower outer, lower inner. The spread of cancer from the breast to other areas of the body is called metastasis. This can happen three ways: through the lymphatic system (lymph nodes and vessels), through the vascular system (blood), or through direct extension from the primary tumor. Tumor size is measured in centimeters. A 1-centimeter lesion has a ⅓-inch diameter, and is about the size of a small pearl. Two and a half centimeters is 1 inch, and 4 centimeters is 1½ inches, or the size of a Ping-Pong ball.

What Are Premalignant Conditions?

All abnormalities of the breast fall into three categories: benign, premalignant, and malignant. Benign lesions or masses do not become cancer. Premalignant conditions, however, can develop into cancer in the near or distant future. These conditions indicate unusual cell activity and often show up on a mammogram but are not yet palpable. They must be treated with the same thoughtfulness as true breast cancers.

Many premalignant conditions are discovered as abnormalities on a mammogram. Most of the time, they are clusters of tiny deposits of calcium in the soft tissue — calcifications — which you cannot feel. Precancerous lesions detected on a mammogram will progress to cancer 10 to 20 percent of the time. One precancerous condition is *atypical hyperplasia* (either ductal or lobular). *Hyperplasia* means the excessive growth of cells. *Atypical* means the cells have characteristics which may develop into cancer. Typically, a single layer of cells lines a duct. With hyperplasia, the lining of the duct is several cell layers thick but the cells are not malignant. When the cells become malignant but are still within the duct, the cancer is *in situ* (in place; that is, it has not broken through to surrounding tissue). If the cells break through the duct lining into surrounding tissue, the cancer is *invasive*. Breast cancer grows over long periods. If these conditions are premalignant, they remain localized, or contained within that area, until they develop into noninvasive cancer or invasive cancer. Then there is the potential for spread into surrounding breast tissue or even the rest of the body. This is one reason early detection is so important.

Lobular carcinoma in situ (LCIS), or lobular neoplasia, is another early sign of potential cancer that appears mostly in *pre*menopausal women. In most cases it is an incidental finding during a biopsy for another abnormality, such as a benign lump. It appears as a change noted in the tissue, abnormal cell growth. Some feel it is not a cancer, and unless it undergoes a change, it cannot metastasize to the rest of your body. The condition is multicentric in 30 percent of women and involves both breasts (bilateral) in 30 to 50 percent of women. It never disappears, but 50 to 70 percent of the time LCIS *does not* progress to cancer, and when it does it may take up to twenty years for the true cancer to evidence.

In the past, this condition was always treated with mastectomy because when mastectomy specimens were examined by the pathologist, multifocal lobular neoplasia (then called lobular carcinoma in situ) was found in 30 to 50 percent of patients. Because the chance of developing breast cancer was high, and because the cancer could potentially develop in more than one area of the breast, mastectomy was usually prescribed. Because it can become cancer, or heralds the development of cancer, women with this diagnosis who find the "watch and wait" method intolerable, have chosen bilateral simple mastectomy and reconstruction as an option. Recently, watch-and-wait or lumpectomy and close follow-up have been offered more frequently as treatment options.

The Multiple Faces of Breast Cancer

In situ and invasive breast cancer. Breast cancer is either in situ or invasive. *In situ* means "in place." The cancer has not broken through the duct wall or lobule into the surrounding tissue. It is *non*invasive. Invasive, or infiltrating, breast cancer has broken through the duct wall into surrounding tissue. It is common to have a combination of in situ and invasive breast cancer. An undetected in situ tumor frequently develops invasive components as it grows. Pockets of in situ or invasive cells can develop in different areas of the same tumor. If the cancer is invasive and larger than 1 centimeter, the size of a small pearl, lymph nodes around the breast and under the arm must be checked to find out if the cancer has begun to spread. Your lymph fluids flow through your body via a network of vessels, the way the bloodstream flows through veins and arteries, and the lymph nodes are like filters, catching what comes through the pipes. As part of the immune system, they filter out foreign or abnormal cells to get rid of them. It is here that breast cancer cells are likely to travel — about 30 percent of the time.

Ductal carcinoma in situ (DCIS). This early breast cancer usually presents as a very small tumor or cluster of calcifications and is localized within the breast ducts. It can be multicentric, however, and is usually associated with microcalcifications. It is detected more and more frequently by mammography. Because the carcinoma has not broken through, or invaded, the wall or lining of the duct (intraductal), lymph node involvement is rare (1–2 percent) and most surgeons don't recommend lymph node dissection *unless* an area over 2 centimeters (¾ inch) is noted. This would increase the possibility of an undetected invasive cancer.

Comedo carcinoma is a type of ductal carcinoma in situ that seems to be more aggressive and to recur locally more frequently. It can occur alone or in combination with invasive carcinoma. Lymph node metastasis is unusual, and in cases where this has happened, it is assumed there was undocumented invasive cancer present. *Papillary carcinoma* is not common and usually is not invasive. Under the microscope, the cells look like fingers projecting into the duct space. Solid tumors have an even pattern of cells throughout the duct, and a *cribriform carcinoma* has a pattern like Swiss cheese. These two types also have a favorable outcome.

Invasive ductal carcinoma. This is the most common breast cancer, and 60 percent of the time it presents as a small, hard tumor or lump. The cancer cells have started to break through the duct wall to the breast tissue outside the duct. Tumors up to 4 centimeters (1½ inches) in diameter can be treated with lumpectomy and radiation therapy. Because this cancer is invasive, lymph nodes are removed at the time of the lumpectomy so they can be checked for cancer cells.

Medullary carcinoma, a variant of invasive ductal carcinoma, represents about 1 percent of breast cancers. This is often a soft gray tumor as large as 5 to 10 centimeters (2–4 inches). Despite its size, it still can be localized in the breast and is less likely than a standard invasive ductal carcinoma to spread to the lymph nodes. *Mucinous* (or colloid) *carcinoma* is an unusual variant of invasive ductal carcinoma that grows slowly over many years and tends to occur in postmenopausal women. The cells produce mucin (the lubricant protecting body surfaces) and the tumor is soft. It often appears in combination with other types of invasive ductal cancers.

Invasive lobular carcinoma. This is similar to invasive ductal carcinoma in its potential to metastasize, but it seems to have a slightly higher potential to become bilateral. Unlike the ductal variety, which presents often as a small, hard lump, this appears as a thickening of the breast. It has spidery extensions into surrounding tissue and can be difficult to detect on mammogram and physical examination.

Inflammatory breast cancer. This rare breast cancer mimics an infection or inflammation and is sometimes misdiagnosed as mastitis and treated with antibiotics. The breast can become swollen and tender, the skin red and warm. The cancer cells invade the lymph system of the skin and block the lymph vessels so that skin can look like an orange peel, a condition called *peau d'orange*. Historically, this breast cancer has a dismal prognosis, but aggressive chemotherapy incorporated into the treatment plan — before and after surgery — and possibly radiation therapy, is improving the picture.

Paget's disease. This rare breast cancer causes a rash resembling eczema on the nipple and areola, or a discharge from the nipple, or sometimes the nipple may actually invert. There is usually an invasive carcinoma in the underlying breast, or ductal carcinoma in situ (DCIS) in the nipple ducts. Mastectomy is still the standard treatment because excision of the nipple alone leaves the breast deformed. But if a mammogram shows no other abnormalities in the rest of the breast and no lump can be felt to suggest a more extensive process, then lumpectomy (removal of the nipple and areola) with radiation therapy usually controls local recurrence. As procedures improve, some surgeons are having good results with nipple reconstruction.

Bilateral breast cancer. About 10 to 15 percent of breast cancer is bilateral — both-sided. It can appear simultaneously (synchronous) or it may appear more than a year later in the second breast (metachronous). One of the most important things for your physician to do if you develop a new cancer in the opposite breast is *rule out that this is a metastasis* from the primary cancer in the first breast. Treatment is different for a metastatic lesion as opposed to a new primary. Each breast must be considered individually.

In the past, bilateral mastectomy was standard, but if both breasts show early-stage disease, with a tumor of less than or equal to 4 to 5 centimeters (about 2 inches) and there is no sign of multifocal disease, then lumpectomy with lymph node dissection and radiation therapy can be offered for both breasts. Radiation can be safely delivered to each breast with no more complications than those described in Chapter 7. If you have multifocal disease in one breast but small limited disease in the other, a lumpectomy and lymph node dissection with radiation can be performed on one side and mastectomy on the other side. Bilateral reconstruction can also be performed.

Axillary adenopathy. An enlarged lymph node under your arm or anywhere around your breast is presumed to be from breast problems even though no breast lump is found. One percent of breast cancers present as enlarged axillary nodes without a palpable breast lump. Axillary lymph nodes can become enlarged from a systemic virus or infection, or an injury to your arm, hand, or breast, as well as from another type of cancer. A mammogram and biopsy must rule out other cancers and multicentric disease because treatment will differ. An X ray or CAT scan may be needed to check for other enlarged nodes, too.

The original breast cancer may never be found — even after mastectomy, when breast tissue is checked under the microscope. It may be so small that the pathologist cannot see it without sectioning the entire breast, and that would be an impossible task. It could also come from an undetected cancer in the opposite breast. Mastectomy and chemotherapy is the most common treatment. Radiation to the entire breast has been used, but this is tricky when the radiation therapist doesn't know exactly where the original breast cancer is and thus where to apply the "boost," the final radiation dose that usually focuses on the site of the tumor.

Lymphomas of the breast. Sometimes a lump in your breast is not breast cancer, but cancer of the lymph system. Lymphoma can cause lymph nodes to enlarge in the axilla and present as a mass in the breast. It can be primary (starting in the lymphatic tissue in the breast) or systemic (the breast mass is only one of the tumors with lymphoma throughout the body). Treatment includes a combination of chemotherapy, surgery, and sometimes radiation.

Sarcomas are rare malignancies that often can be locally aggressive and can occasionally metastasize widely. They are large, fleshy masses that grow in the connective tissue (collagen) of the breast. Because they can grow to be so big, they cause the breast to enlarge and appear distorted. For this reason they are usually treated with mastectomy. A variety of sarcomas can arise from different parts of the breast. For instance, angiosarcoma originates in blood vessels; liposarcoma, in fat cells; leiomyosarcoma, in the smooth muscle cells; and rhabdomyosarcoma, in the structured muscle cells. They can arise in the breast, or metastasize from a sarcoma elsewhere in the body. This is very different from cystosarcoma, which is one of the least aggressive sarcomas.

Male breast cancer. One percent of all breast cancers appear in men. Because men don't suspect breast cancer, tumors tend to be diagnosed at a more advanced stage. Treatment options include mastectomy or lumpectomy with radiation. Because this book is written for women, we have not expounded on the treatment of male breast cancer.

~ 2

Where to Get a Reliable and Safe Mammogram

Mammography has an exceedingly important role to play in the diagnosis, evaluation, and aftercare of breast cancer. No other radiological tool is yet as useful in finding out what is going on in the breast. Even though mammograms can miss 10 to 15 percent of breast tumors, they are safe and highly accurate when they are done right. As of October 1994, all mammography facilities are required to have accreditation from the American College of Radiology (ACR). This accreditation lets you know that the radiologists are specially trained and certified in mammography and that the equipment meets certain standards and is inspected annually. The technicians are also specially trained. Before this federal regulation, fewer than half the mammography facilities in the United States had ACR accreditation.

Some diagnostic centers do all kinds of X rays and may spend only a small part of their time performing and reading mammograms. Ask how many mammograms are performed at the facility you are considering. You should expect a reliable reading from a facility that evaluates at least fifteen to thirty mammograms a day. A breast imaging center in a major medical facility will perform a hundred or more each day. Also ask if the center uses the *film screen method* of mammography, which uses less radiation and is easier to interpret than the older xeromammograms, which are printed on paper.

Over the past twenty years the dose of radiation required for mammography has been dramatically reduced with improved film, equipment, and technology. A mammogram is now a low-energy X ray, and the most up-to-date mammographic equipment delivers only one-tenth of a rad — the unit of measure for radiation — to each breast. This is less than a standard chest X ray.

Look for a facility that can do ultrasound or take supplemental views of your breast the same day if necessary to get a more precise picture. Magnified pictures or pictures from different angles are sometimes needed to get a better look at an area that is not clearly defined in the mammogram. Ultrasound can often clarify whether a mass is solid or fluid-filled. Before you go, find out if it is the policy of the facility to give you the results after your films are studied. A radiologist — a medical doctor who specializes in diagnosis through X rays and is certified in radiology — will speak with you after your films are taken. Avoid any place that won't tell you anything until they talk with your physician — unless your physician requested this for some reason. You could spend days in a state of anxiety. For this same reason, avoid going on Friday if you can. Ask your doctor ahead of time to be sure he or she has no objections to the radiologist's discussing the results with you.

What Your Mammography Workup Includes

A standard mammographic workup includes two views of each breast from different angles. Additional views and breast ultrasound will be obtained if needed. The procedure itself takes about five minutes. If you have a lump in one breast, you must get pictures of both breasts, so they can be compared, and also to check the other breast for any abnormalities. If you have had a mammogram before, the radiologist will use the old one as a baseline for comparison. Don't wear powders or deodorant with talcum when you go. Talcum can mimic breast calcifications in mammography.

Why Proper Compression Is So Important

Because your breast is squeezed flat between two metal or plastic plates for a few seconds, getting a mammogram can hurt. But proper compression is *essential* to get the lowest radiation dose and highest-quality mammogram. All of your breast tissue must be pulled forward, away from your chest wall, so it can be included in the picture. Women who are very young, or who have dense breasts, can present a problem. Here's where the technician's ability and training count. Compression may hurt more if you are premenstrual and your breasts are engorged and tender. Consider this when you make the appointment. If you have a breast implant, find out if the technician knows the Ecklund technique of compression, which images as much breast tissue as possible and prevents the implant from being X-rayed.

Why Additional Views Are Needed

Additional compression views and magnification are often needed to try to better evaluate tiny lesions or calcifications. Sometimes a lesion that is very high or in the lower fold (inframammary) of the breast or near the center of the breast can be missed if the breast is too small to get the lump on the film. Angled views are needed to check these areas.

How Mammograms Are Interpreted

Mammography is not an exact science. Much depends on the interpretation and experience of the radiologist. Both benign and malignant tumors can show up as calcifications, masses, or densities on a mammogram, so it may be impossible to make a precise determination. That's why it is so important to have an experienced radiologist reading your films. Lesions can be benign, indeterminate, or suspicious, depending on the pattern, clustering, shape, size, and configuration.

Ideally, the radiologist should review your films and tell you what shows up. Some may want to tell you as little as possible because they prefer talking with your physician, or have been instructed not to tell you. But you have a right to know. Try to look at the films with the radiologist and ask specific questions about shape, size, or other characteristics: "What is it you see?" "Where is it?" "What do you think it could be?" Remember, the radiologist does not know your full history and may defer a final decision for other tests to your primary doctor or surgeon.

Finding a Reliable Mammography Facility

To find an accredited breast imaging center in your area, ask your doctor or call one of the breast cancer information hotlines (see Appendix 4). Also check local women's health networks. The human resources department where you work may be helpful as well. And please, if it means the difference between traveling some distance for a proper mammogram or getting one at a questionable facility close by, take the trip! Take someone — and your notebook — with you.

What Mammograms Cost

Mammograms cost between $100 and $200; usually $50 to $100 for the film and technology, and an equal amount for the interpretation by the radiologist. Most medical insurance now covers mammography when it is part of a diagnostic workup, but routine preventive screenings are not always covered. Check your health insurance plan to see what is provided for screenings.

Free or very low cost mammograms are often available

through community groups, local businesses, or hospitals. These facilities are less likely to provide all of the services such as magnification views or immediate ultrasound follow-up and interpretation. Many corporations now provide free or low-cost mammograms and classes in breast self-examination to their employees and to women in the community.

By the way, your X rays are yours, part of your medical records. You can take them with you to show your doctors or just to keep if you want. If you move to another region, you should take them with you. This will save time when you need them for comparison in a new place. *Just don't lose them.* Store them flat in a dry place.

Other Breast Imaging Techniques

Because 10 to 15 percent of breast cancer and lumps do not show up on mammography, other techniques for seeing into your breasts may be necessary to evaluate a mass or density you discovered through physical examination.

Ultrasound converts sound waves bouncing off your breast tissue into images on a screen. This is a very noninvasive test and does not expose you to radiation. A handheld transducer, or probe, scans your breast and sends images to the screen. Ultrasound can often supplement mammography and determine if a lesion is solid or cystic. A cyst is fluid-filled and looks like a water balloon. It appears smooth and black on the ultrasound screen. Solid masses appear gray but not the same gray as the surrounding tissue. Ultrasound is also one of the most sensitive ways to evaluate the integrity of a breast implant, to be certain there has not been a leak.

CAT (or CT) scan. CAT stands for "computerized axial tomography." While you lie inside a wide tube, this X ray translates information into two-dimensional "slices," or cross sections. This is an excellent way to look at your chest wall, lungs, and lymph node–bearing areas around your collarbone, under your arm, and between your chest wall and lungs. A surgeon may use this to see if a deep lesion is attached to the chest wall. Computed tomography can also be used to evaluate the lungs, liver, abdomen, and pelvis for signs of metastasis. The radiation dose from a CAT scan is considerably higher than that from a routine mammogram. The amount depends on the number of "slices" needed and on the part of the body being scanned. CAT scan is used in planning radiation treatment to outline the field, or area, to be treated.

MRI (magnetic resonance imaging). Because it is costly and less specific than mammography, MRI is generally not used to screen for breast cancer. Like a CAT scan, it can give a better image of the chest wall, lungs, and nodal groups. Together with ultrasound, it is the best way to evaluate silicone breast implants for rupture. Scientists are developing the MRI capability to differentiate between malignant and benign breast processes and to evaluate lymph nodes for metastasis. Patients are often afraid of the procedure because it means being confined in a long tube for as much as an hour. However, a mild sedative makes most claustrophobic patients relax.

Transillumination. This technique works by shining low-intensity red or near-infrared light through the breast. It is not used often because its accuracy rate is low.

Thermography measures heat, in effect taking the temperature of the cancer site. Cancers are thought to have more blood flow than normal tissue; this makes them warmer, and so they appear as "hot spots" on a thermographic "map" of the breast. In the past, thermography was used to find superficial lesions. It was not very sensitive and was used when nothing else was available. It is rarely used today.

✔ Questions to Ask About a Mammography
Facility

These questions are meant to help you interview physicians and other healthcare professionals so that you can feel secure about your treatment decisions. Some of these questions have no clear-cut answers, some do. But ask anyway!

When were you accredited for mammography by the American College of Radiology?

As of October 1994, all mammography centers in the United States had to have this certification to stay in business. It lets you know they have regulated and annually inspected equipment and properly trained radiologists.

Is a certified radiologist available to talk with me right after my films are reviewed?

You want a radiologist who is experienced at reading mammograms, because many benign and malignant lesions can look similar. If the radiologist can tell you the findings the day the X rays are taken, you won't go home without knowing anything. Be certain that your doctor has given the radiologist permission to discuss the findings with you.

Is the technician certified in mammography?

The X-ray technician needs training to compress your breast properly so that the mammogram is as accurate as possible. Certification also assures that the technologist knows how to position you properly for special views and get acceptable pictures. Radiology technicians are certified by the American Registry of Radiology Technicians. If they take special training in mammography, they are subcertified in mammography by that national organization. As of 1995, the American College of Radiology requires technicians to be certified as part of the accreditation requirements for a mammography facility.

How many mammograms are done here every day?

If you are at a comprehensive breast imaging or cancer center, or an academic medical center in a large city, you can expect the staff to read hundreds of mammograms a month. In any case, you want to go where they see fifteen or more mammograms a day.

Do you use the film screen method of mammography?

This method is preferred over the older xeromammogram type because it uses less radiation and is more accurate.

Will you forward my films as well as my report to physicians if I request?

Your other physicians will probably rely on oral and written reports from the radiologist, because surgeons or other specialists may be less experienced in interpreting the films. But some surgeons or other specialists may want to see your films personally, particularly if there is a change on a new mammogram.

May I take the films with me today?

You bought them, you can take them with you. They are part of your medical records, and you should be able to show them to other doctors if you are relocating or getting additional opinions. You will need them for comparison when you have mammograms in the future. (Store them flat in a dry place.)

What is the total cost? Is there a charge for additional views?

Total cost — for film and consultation — should be between $100 and $200. Most insurance coverage includes mammography when it is part of the diagnostic process. Additional views or ultrasound may add to the cost.

What exactly do you see? Where is it?

If there is an abnormality or change from your previous mammogram, ask the radiologist to point out what the film shows, such as a lesion in the lower outer quadrant of the breast. Ask about the shape, size, characteristics, whether it looks like a cyst or solid tumor or calcifications. The radiologist may tell you what he or she thinks it is and also suggest further testing, such as ultrasound, CAT scan, or biopsy.

When will my physician have this information?
The same day, if verbal reports are provided by phone. Certainly by the next day, unless it's 5 P.M. on Friday. Written reports take three to five days to get to your doctor. Ask if you can deliver the report yourself.

~ 3

What Your Biopsy
Will Tell You

Before a treatment plan can be outlined, your breast tumor must be studied under a microscope to determine its type, size, and cell activity. Sometimes a biopsy can be done by inserting a needle into the tumor and pulling out some of the cells to see if they are cancerous. This is often used as a preliminary step, but the surgical biopsy, which removes part or all of the abnormality, is the most commonly used because it gives us a chance to get the most information — with our own eyes and under a microscope — about what is going on. This biopsy may be the first of several histologic studies. After a lumpectomy and lymph node dissection, or a mastectomy, more breast tissue and lymph nodes will be studied to gather further information about your breast cancer.

What's Involved in a Surgical Biopsy?

Most surgical biopsies are now done as an outpatient procedure with local anesthesia to numb the breast. You may also receive some intravenous sedation that will wear off in twenty to thirty minutes. Surgery will take fifteen to thirty minutes, but you may be at the surgical center longer for a needle-guided or ultrasound-guided biopsy. These procedures require some time for the X ray or ultrasound to locate the area to be biopsied. From the time you arrive until you go home is two to three hours.

Informed consent. You will be asked to sign consent forms for anesthesia, biopsy, and for every procedure you encounter from now on. Don't sign anything until you know exactly what will happen. This is what "informed consent" means. (We will talk more about this in the chapter on surgery.) Let the doctors know about any medications you are using. Ask what kind of anesthesia they plan to use, how it will affect you, and what aftereffects it will have. Write the answers down. Some typical drugs used are lidocaine or Xylocaine for locally numbing your breast, and intravenous Valium (diazepam) or Versed (midazolam) for relaxing or sedating you. Because you may be weakened or drowsy from intravenous anesthesia, you may also have to promise that someone will take you home if you receive anything but local anesthesia.

Pretesting Before Surgical Biopsy. Before a surgical biopsy, you may be scheduled for preoperative tests such as a chest X ray, an EKG (electrocardiogram), and blood tests to check your general health and be sure you are able to tolerate surgery and regional or general anesthesia. If only local anesthesia will be used, you may not get these tests. You may also speak with the anesthesiologist at this time.

Surgery. Once you have changed into a hospital gown and cap, you will probably walk with the anesthesiologist into the operating room. If you were injected with intravenous sedation, you should feel relaxed. The anesthesiologist and one or more nurses and surgical residents are in the room with you and your surgeon. You may be awake and able to talk throughout the procedure, but you will not feel any pain. You can also ask to see the piece of tissue taken from your breast.

Most common incision locations are at the areolar margin or directly over the lesion. The abnormal area will be dissected away from the normal tissue and removed. Surgeons experienced with breast cancer can often identify the lesion when they see it, except for smaller lesions like calcifications. A surgical biopsy will remove a sample of your tumor (incisional), or, if your tumor is a small one, the entire lesion will probably be taken out (excisional). Most lesions smaller than 3 centimeters (1 inch) will be removed completely at the time of the biopsy.

The excised tissue is sent to the pathologist for immediate evaluation to see if cancer is present. This is done by freezing a piece of the tissue and is known as a frozen section. Ask your surgeon if a frozen section will be done. If the abnormality is too small or too diffuse, frozen section may not be possible, and you will have to wait a few days for the results of the biopsy.

The biopsy area will be cauterized to control bleeding and your incision will be closed up, sutured, or stitched. A short piece of latex tube may extend from the wound to allow any excess fluids to drain out. A soft wad of gauze to cover your incision will be held in place with something like an Ace bandage wrapped around your chest.

You will rest in the recovery room for about an hour, until your doctor is certain that you have tolerated the procedure and anesthesia and there is no bleeding. And — most important — until the preliminary pathology report from the frozen section is available and you learn whether or not you have cancer. This will be an anxious time, no doubt about it. Although a frozen section is 95 to 98 percent accurate, if the result is not clear, your surgeon may prefer to wait for the full report. This is often referred to as the permanent section — the entire piece of tissue removed will be permanently "fixed" to allow for a full histologic study. It is better to wait a few days for the correct answer than rush and get a wrong diagnosis. Before you are sent home, you will be given something to eat and drink, probably crackers and tea or juice. Instructions for home care should come from your surgeon or the nursing staff before you leave the surgical center.

Follow-up care. The next day, when you remove your dressing, the tube will fall out by itself. You can shower and pat dry the incision. It might be comfortable to keep it covered by sticking fresh gauze pads inside your bra. If you don't wear a bra, lightly tape the gauze pad in place, but tape may irritate your skin. You may be more comfortable wearing a bra twenty-four hours a day for about a week so the weight of your breast does not put stress on the wound.

A few days or a week later, your surgeon will examine your wound and discuss your full biopsy report with you in detail. At this point there may be a telephone conference with your treatment team.

Needle-guided biopsy. This is a surgical biopsy and is usually called for when no lump is palpable but calcifications or microscopic lesions show up on a mammogram. The procedure begins in the mammography area (assuming you are in a medical center), where the radiologist looks at your films and inserts a long needle through your breast to the site of the abnormality. A wire may also be placed with or through the needle. This sounds much worse than it feels. Surprisingly, it does not hurt much. Another mammogram then confirms the correct position of the needle. Then in the operating room the surgeon makes the incision near the needle. Tissue is removed from your breast and is usually X-rayed while you are on the operating table to confirm that the suspicious lesion has been removed. This is a specimen X ray. If the lesion is not seen in the specimen X rays, the surgeon can remove more tissue if necessary.

If the surgeon can't find the lesions, the incision is closed and dressed as with the other biopsy. You'll have to get another mammogram in two or three months when your scar heals and the postsurgical swelling of your breast tissue recedes. If your follow-up mammogram shows nothing, the calcifications have either dissolved on their own or they were removed by the surgeon but were undetected by the specimen X ray at the time of surgery. About 25 to 30 percent of needle-guided biopsies will reveal a cancer and up to half of these will be in situ disease.

Ultrasound-guided biopsy. Ultrasound guides the surgeon the same way as the needle-guided biopsy. Before surgery the breast is scanned with the ultrasound and the skin over the lesion is marked with a felt-tip pen. Once the abnormality is removed, another ultrasound scan confirms that the suspicious lesion is gone. If necessary, ultrasound can be performed during the surgery to direct the surgeon to the abnormality.

When Nonsurgical Biopsy Is Performed

Some lumps or abnormalities can be evaluated without a surgical biopsy.

Fine-needle aspiration biopsy (needle cytology) is often a first step when evaluating a lump to try to see if it is fluid-filled or solid. This procedure is usually done in the doctor's office. Using a syringe and needle, the doctor extracts some fluid or cells from the lesion and sends it to a cytopathologist for testing to determine if malignant cells are present. The results are 90 to 95 percent accurate and it is less expensive than surgical biopsy. But the sample is smaller and is more difficult to interpret than a piece of tissue under a microscope.

Stereotactic core biopsy. This newly developed technique — which takes only twenty minutes — can determine whether a tiny lesion detected only through mammography is cancerous or not. While you lie facedown on a table, your breast hangs through a hole. A revolving mammography unit attached to the underside of the table rotates to obtain three-dimensional images of your breast from several angles. The exact location of the lesion is calculated by a computer.

After your breast is anesthetized and you are still in the facedown position, the radiologist uses a hollow-core needle to retrieve five inch-long, cylinder-shaped samples of tissue from the area of the lesion. Accuracy demands that cells removed be examined by a cytopathologist, an expert in interpreting cellular samples. This requires more exacting interpretation than tissue from a surgical biopsy, but it can be a way to avoid surgical biopsy, which is more expensive. If there is any question about the results, a surgical biopsy is performed, usually a needle-guided biopsy. The equipment and expertise for stereotactic core biopsy is available at large medical centers.

What You Can Learn from Your Pathology Report

Surprisingly few women ask any questions about their pathology report. All women should. This report gives you information you need to make the best treatment choices, and you should become familiar with it. Ask your surgeon to tell you what everything in the report means. Take it with you when you talk with other doctors for additional opinions.

When the pathologist studies the tiny piece of tissue on your slide under the microscope, many things about your cancer are revealed. The tumor size is measured, and the margins of the piece of tissue are checked to see if your tumor extends to the edges. If the entire tumor is removed, it can be easily measured. If only a piece is removed, measurement can be calculated from what the surgeon saw as well as what shows up on the mammogram. The tumor cells are examined to determine if they are invasive, how fast they are growing, how aggressive they are. If your cancer is invasive, further tests will be done. These pieces of information — the variables of breast cancer — are called prognostic indicators. They help guide you and your doctors with decision making about treatment.

For instance, the pathologist may look for necrosis — dead

tumor tissue — which could indicate a fast-growing tumor that has outgrown its blood supply. Or inflammatory cells may be found around the tumor, which could mean your immune system is already fighting the cancer. Because there is still so much we don't know about breast cancer, we rely heavily on what we *do* know, so the more information we have, the better. Among the items typically found on a pathology report are the following:

Estrogen and progesterone receptor (ER/PR) analysis. Estrogen receptors and progesterone receptors are proteins on the outside wall of the cancer cell. Tumors *with* hormone receptors are most like normal cells and generally grow more slowly and are less likely to spread. The presence or absence of these receptors indicates how you may respond to chemotherapy or hormone treatment. For instance, if your report is positive for estrogen receptors, you would most likely benefit from hormone therapy, such as tamoxifen, which is directed at blocking estrogen. The tamoxifen binds with the receptor and prevents estrogen from getting into any residual cancer cells. If the tumor is negative for hormone receptors, you may be a candidate for cytotoxic chemotherapy (that is, drugs intended to destroy or slow down the cancer cells), depending on the other factors of your diagnosis.

Margins of resection. You will frequently hear the term "clean" (or "clear") "margins." Clean margins mean there is a cancer-free border around your tumor on the tissue removed from your breast. This information is critical in determining your candidacy for radiation therapy. The rate of recurrence in the breast may be greater if you do not have clear margins, but this depends on how much disease there is at the margins. If your tumor was removed piecemeal, or the surgeon was able to see that not all the disease was removed, then the information on margins is less specific. If the cancer appears too diffuse, then radiation and lumpectomy may not be an option, even if you have a small tumor.

Grade looks at the overall pattern of the tumor cells and nuclei. It also lets us know how aggressive the cancer is. Grade I describes the least aggressive form, Grade III the most aggressive — and the most common. There is also a nuclear grade, which classifies individual cells for bland (less aggressive) or bizarre (more aggressive) nuclei.

Flow cytometry determines your "S phase fraction," the number of cancer cells actively multiplying, or synthesizing. A tumor with a high percentage in the S phase of the cell cycle is usually more aggressive. This information can help determine the use of chemotherapy.

DNA analysis also helps determine how aggressive your cancer is. If a normal complement of DNA is found in the nucleus of a cell, it is labeled *diploid* and the cancer may be less aggressive. If cells contain less or more than a normal amount of DNA, the tumor is *aneuploid* and therefore more aggressive. The DNA index for a diploid tumor is 1.00, so any number higher or lower than that indicates an aneuploid tumor.

Other studies are still considered investigational but are used increasingly to fine-tune treatment options, especially in choosing medication for chemotherapy. Angiogenesis, the ability of the tumor to grow blood vessels, gives us a clue to the speed of metastasis, and so the number of blood vessels in the tumor are counted. Cathepsin D is an enzyme, and it has been noted that tumors high in this enzyme are more aggressive. HER-2/neu, a type of gene associated with tumor formation, is a genetic factor that might indicate the risk of recurrence. Ki 67 evaluates the nuclear proliferation antigen and would be high with rapidly growing tumors. MDR-1, the multiple drug resistance gene, might provide information on how well chemotherapy would work. Transformed cells contain more p53 (mutated gene) than normal cells, and rapidly dividing cells contain more p53 than stationary cells, so we look for high expression of this to indicate more aggressive tumors.

The Second Biopsy: Lymph Node Status

Another critical component of your diagnosis is the status of
your lymph nodes. Are they negative or positive for cancer?
If your original biopsy reveals invasive cancer, some of your
axillary (underarm) lymph nodes are removed surgically and
analyzed at the time of your lumpectomy or mastectomy. This
surgery is known as axillary dissection, and we describe the
entire procedure in Chapter 5.

There are lymph nodes throughout your body. Those under
your arm on the side with the affected breast are early indicators of whether or not cancer has spread from your breast.
Any lymph node showing cancer is evaluated to see if the
cancer is contained inside the node or has broken through the
shell of the node. A pathologist may examine from ten to fifty
lymph nodes, depending on how thorough a dissection is
performed and how many nodes you have.

What a Biopsy Costs

Most medical insurance covers biopsy procedure and pathology, or laboratory tests, but maybe not all. Tests will cost
several hundred dollars. You should check your insurance first.
Be sure that the particular pathology lab you are planning to
use accepts your medical insurance. If not, discuss this with
your surgeon and find out what other alternative you have.
You may be able to negotiate a reduced charge if your surgeon
wants to use that particular lab.

Can I Get a Second Opinion?

The pathologist and laboratory are usually chosen by your
surgeon or hospital, and rarely are you asked if you would like
to choose your own pathology lab! You can get another pathology opinion, though. Your pathology slides are part of your

medical records and you can take them to another pathologist. Hospital laboratories keep these tissue samples for many years. You will probably have to give the laboratory twenty-four hours' notice in writing, or sign a hospital form so the lab can release the slides and a written report.

✔ Questions to Ask About Your Pathology Reports

These questions are meant to help you interview physicians and other healthcare professionals so that you can feel secure about your treatment decisions. Some of these questions have no clear-cut answers, some do. But ask anyway!

How long will it take to get the complete pathology results?

It should take two to three days maximum, but most surgeons discuss results with you when you go back to the office for a postbiopsy checkup in a week. Some special test results, like the DNA analysis, are sometimes sent to specialized laboratories and it may be two weeks or more before you have results.

What type of tumor do I have?

You want to know if it is premalignant or a true cancer and whether it is invasive or in situ, ductal or lobular. Ask for a description of its characteristics. Is it an aggressive or slow-growing tumor?

How big is it, and where is it?

Size is measured in centimeters, so ask how that translates into inches. Is it centrally located or in one quadrant of the breast? Which quadrant? Is the nipple or areola involved?

Is it multicentric or multifocal?

You want to know if your tumor is isolated, or whether there are other lesions in your breast. If there is more than one lesion in the same quadrant of your breast, your cancer is multifocal. If lesions are detected in other quadrants of your breast, it is multicentric.

Do I have clean margins?

If you had a surgical biopsy, the area around the tumor site — the margin — is either clean, meaning cancer free, or it shows spidery extensions into the edges of the specimen tissue. This is important in determining if you are a candidate for lumpectomy, axillary dissection, and radiation.

How aggressive is the cancer?

The grade and DNA analysis of your cancer can provide this information. Grade I is least aggressive, and Grade III is most aggressive. The DNA index tells you whether it is diploid (slow-growing) or aneuploid (fast-growing).

Do I have positive or negative hormone receptors?

This is usually measured as the percentage of cells showing estrogen receptors and progesterone receptors. For example, a report may indicate: ER 75 percent, PR 5 percent. Some laboratories report the results in absolute numbers. You are considered to have positive receptors with a higher number, or percentage, and negative receptors with lower numbers. The status of your receptors affects options for tamoxifen or other chemotherapy.

What do my lymph nodes show?

If you had an axillary dissection, you should find out how many lymph nodes are positive, whether the cancer is breaking through the capsule (outer skin of the node), whether the entire node is involved or only a microscopic part.

If I want a second pathologist's opinion, how long will it take to get my slides from the pathology department?

You should be able to get your slides within twenty-four hours. You will have to sign them out of the lab. You need to call the day before to give the pathology department time to get the slides ready along with a typed report.

～ 4

After the Biopsy:
How Much Time to Make Decisions?

Now you know what kind of breast cancer you have and
whether or not it's invasive, but you don't have the complete
picture yet. The remaining evaluation and staging — for invasive breast cancer — cannot be done until after surgery,
when lymph nodes can be removed and analyzed. If some
nodes show cancer, more tests may be necessary before your
workup is complete.

Nevertheless, you have to make some decisions now. Do
you want a lumpectomy or mastectomy? Will you need chemotherapy? What kind of local treatment should you have before
you know if you need systemic treatment? Local treatment
includes surgery and radiation. Systemic treatment is chemotherapy and bone marrow transplantation.

It is quite likely that the surgeon who does your biopsy will
recommend the best treatment, whether you have a premalignant condition, like lobular neoplasia, or a true cancer. Try to
begin treatment within three or four weeks of diagnosis, but
don't be rushed. Now is the time to get all the information
and support you need, as well as a second or third opinion.
Avoid getting the second opinion in the same hospital or
medical center, where thinking may be uniform. To find other

breast cancer specialists, you can turn to the resources in the back of the book.

Go with an open mind. Other physicians will review your workup and evaluation, confirm the diagnosis, and discuss available options with you. Each time you speak to someone you'll learn more; it may take several conferences to get a grasp of the situation. You are extremely vulnerable now, so try to remain objective. Bring someone along for moral support. Don't forget your notebook.

Completing Your Workup

If you have been diagnosed with invasive breast cancer, or you have positive lymph nodes, you may be given additional tests to be sure your cancer has not metastasized.

An X ray or CAT scan of the chest to look for possible metastasis to the lungs.

Blood tests. Certain blood tests called tumor markers detect metastasis, especially in the liver and bone. CA15-3 looks for breast and ovarian cancer cells; CEA most commonly for colon, lung, and liver cancer cells, but also for breast cancer; CA125 for ovarian cancer and for breast cancer recurrence.

Bone scan. A bone scan checks your entire skeletal system for metastatic deposits. A radioactive isotope (technitium) is injected into your blood and absorbed into your bone. The scanner detects the radiation absorbed in your bone, and areas of increased activity are hotter or appear blacker on the scan. A lesion has to be greater than 1 to 2 centimeters (about ½ inch) to show up on the scan. While only 2 to 3 percent of women with small tumors, or Stage I cancer (see the discussion of staging, below), will have bone metastasis, it can be ruled out early with a bone scan. However, because bone scans are so expensive and not 100 percent accurate, some doctors won't prescribe one unless your risk is high. It is usually prescribed if you have Stage II or higher invasive breast cancer. Regular X rays of the bone, or, ultimately, an MRI (magnetic resonance imaging), may be recommended to further evaluate an abnormal area on the bone scan.

How Breast Cancer Is Staged

Once the mammogram and biopsies, including lymph nodes, have been completed, your breast cancer can be "staged." Staging is based on the clinical examination (clinical stage) and pathological findings (pathological stage). This is a rather elaborate classification system based on the sum of all variables — most important the so-called TNM factors: tumor, nodes, metastasis. Everything your doctors have learned about your breast cancer, from its physical appearance through all the tests, is classified and subclassified; this includes size, type, and location of tumor, and whether or not it is invasive. Staging also considers whether or not the tumor is stuck to the chest wall. The stage of your breast cancer, as well as your general health and personal preferences, helps determine your treatment options. There are subdivisions in the system, such as Stages IIA, IIB, and so on, but generally, the stages can be summed up this way:

- Stage I means the cancer is early and localized to the breast. A primary tumor is less than 2 centimeters (¾ inch), and lymph nodes are not involved.
- Stage II means the tumor is 2 to 5 centimeters (¾ inch– 2 inches) in the breast, or there is evidence of lymph node involvement.
- Stage III means the cancer is locally advanced. The tumor is over 5 centimeters, and/or it has spread to the lymph nodes, or it is inflammatory, but there is no evidence of distant metastasis.
- Stage IV identifies metastatic disease.

There is also a Stage 0 classification, which usually indicates ductal carcinoma in situ with no palpable mass.

Finding Out About Available Treatment Options

Now you are becoming an informed patient. You know what kind of cancer you have, you know what is in your pathology report, and you know the stage of your breast cancer. When you talk with doctors you will understand what treatment involves. There are local treatments such as surgery and radiation directed at the breast and axilla, and systemic treatments such as chemotherapy, which treats the entire body. Let your doctors know you want the truth, not reassurance, no matter how comforting that may seem. Taking charge of your breast cancer is the only way you can feel confident that you are doing all the right things to treat it. Don't lose track of the *goal of treatment*, which is to treat your breast cancer and recover.

Write down questions as you think of them. *There is no such thing as a dumb question* when your health is on the line. Keep track of the information you gather. It's perfectly okay to bring a tape recorder and a notebook to appointments with your doctors. This will help you remember the answers given and allow you to compare opinions and options intelligently. This is a cram course with a whole new language and set of information to absorb quickly. Some physicians may find a tape recorder distracting, but if you discuss it with them first, they often will not mind.

Most people know very little about breast cancer, and it can be devastating news to a family. They will think the worst, that they will lose you. Many women try to protect their families from the details, but this makes everyone's anxiety worse. Talk openly and honestly with your family and friends and especially your children. They will sense your concern and fear if you try to deny it. Explain what is going on so they don't hear it from others, who may be misinformed. People close to you may feel helpless when they cannot do anything to help or fix the situation. Be specific about what you need people to do for you. Now that there is more activism about breast cancer, there's a growing network of information and support — for you and your family.

✔ **Questions to Ask About Treatment Facilities**

These questions are meant to help you interview physicians and other healthcare professionals so that you can feel secure about your treatment decisions. Some of these questions have no clear-cut answers, some do. But ask anyway!

Of all Stage I and II patients at this facility, how many are treated with mastectomy?

It's still common for mastectomy to be the surgery of choice in most of the country, but this is changing as knowledge and sophistication of technique become more widespread. In the Northeast only 25 percent of Stage I and Stage II patients receive mastectomies, while in the Midwest that figure is 75 percent. Physicians' preference will strongly influence practice patterns in some areas.

Is there a multidisciplinary cancer treatment team at the facility?

Many medical centers have multidisciplinary treatment teams for specific diseases. Find out if there is a breast cancer treatment team — often called a breast cancer conference — at the facility. This means you could find a surgeon, radiation oncologist, and medical oncologist, as well as other care providers, who work together in patient care. The formal "team" structure may not be present at all medical centers, but if all the specialties are there you could expect them to work together.

Do you have a radiation therapy facility here?

Radiation therapy requires you to report for treatment five days a week for six to eight weeks. If the facility does not have a radiation treatment center, find out where its patients go. This could mean traveling, and you need to know what is logistically possible to get the best surgery and the best radiation therapy.

Can reconstruction be done at the same time as the mastectomy?
The plastic surgeon should be able to work with the breast
surgeon so that reconstruction begins at the same time as the
mastectomy. (See Chapter 6 on reconstruction.) This is an
extended and complex procedure, and smaller hospitals may
not have as much experience with it. You need to explore
alternatives thoroughly with your surgeons before you decide.

Do you have support systems for breast patients?
Many hospitals have clinical nurse specialists who specialize
in breast cancer. They teach you how to care for yourself when
you get home and recommend support groups, physical therapy, and anything else you need. Written materials are available to you and perhaps videos to take home. Hospital social
workers assist with finding support groups, or programs to help
families make the adjustments they need. Nutritionists and
physical therapists are available in larger medical centers, and
biofeedback counselors are increasingly found on the staffs of
many comprehensive cancer centers.

How long will I remain in the hospital?
For a lumpectomy and lymph node dissection, you are hospitalized overnight; for a mastectomy, two or three days. Breast
reconstructive surgery requires three to four days.

What are the charges?
Always ask what you will be charged for treatment. In addition to the surgeon's fee and hospital room charges, there are
costs for use of the operating room, anesthesia, recovery room,
medications, and an assortment of miscellaneous charges. A
hospital should be able to give you a list of standard charges
for any procedure. You may be asked to sign a consent form,
agreeing to pay charges not covered by insurance. Ask what
these charges are, so you are not surprised later.

What insurance coverage do you accept?

Be sure to check this. Also, be sure your medical insurance does not require a second opinion before it will cover any surgery. Patients sometimes are not aware of this and may be surprised when the bill is not paid by the insurance company.

Treatment:
Know Your Options

～ 5

Surgery: Lumpectomy, Mastectomy, Axillary Dissection

Until recently, there was only one way to treat breast cancer. Amputate the breast. Now we know that we don't always need to do that. Breast conservation — taking out only the lump and some lymph nodes — followed by radiation therapy is just as effective in many cases. It actually mimics mastectomy in that it treats the entire breast. This is not a new idea. Lumpectomy with radiation therapy has been around for thirty years, but only recently has it become more widely accepted.

Changing Attitudes About Breast Cancer Surgery

As more and more women show the same survival rate, along with good local control of the disease, the merits of breast conservation are gaining greater acceptance. Some geographic and physician biases still exist. Lumpectomy is offered to women in the Northeast more readily than to women in the South and Midwest. Twice as often, as a matter of fact. For instance, clinical studies done in the late 1980s showed that in Massachusetts, 21 percent of Medicare patients had breast-conserving surgery compared with only 3.5 percent in Kentucky. A report on this study, released in 1992, showed doctors *and* patients were often still reluctant to believe the treatments were equal.

Elderly women tend to be offered mastectomy much more than breast conservation and radiation; this seems to arise from the idea that seven weeks of radiation would be too much for them, or that they are less interested in keeping their breast. Given the option, many elderly women would still want to preserve their breast if possible. They don't necessarily view seven weeks of radiation as any more inconvenient than undergoing major surgery for mastectomy. Women with limited financial resources often come up against the same assumptions, that they cannot afford to take the time off from work or home to come every day for extended treatment.

Nineteen states have informed consent laws regarding breast cancer. Essentially, these laws mandate that women must be offered treatment options other than mastectomy. However, the comprehensiveness of these rulings varies from state to state. For instance, in New Jersey, informed consent means only that you give the doctor permission to do a biopsy — along with your permission to go ahead and perform any operation necessary if your tumor is malignant. This is not far removed from no consent at all, when a woman could go into an operating room for a biopsy and come out without her breast. In contrast, the Kansas law requires physicians to inform patients of all alternative possibilities, including surgery, radiation, and chemotherapy. These states have informed consent laws for breast cancer treatment:

California	Louisiana	New Jersey
Florida	Maine	New York
Georgia	Maryland	Pennsylvania
Hawaii	Massachusetts	Texas
Illinois	Michigan	Virginia
Kansas	Minnesota	Wisconsin
Kentucky		

The law is defined differently in each state, but Pennsylvania and Virginia have weak informed consent laws, similar to those of New Jersey. Other states may have enacted such legislation since this book was written. If your state does not have an informed consent law, be sure you ask your doctors exactly what they are planning to do. And sign a consent only for that procedure. Do not accept mastectomy as the only possibility until all other treatment options have been thoroughly explained and ruled out.

Lumpectomy or Mastectomy for Early Breast Cancer?

Until the late 1980s, lobular carcinoma in situ (LCIS) was treated by mastectomy, because multifocal and multicentric disease was documented in 30 to 50 percent of patients. *Multifocal*, remember, indicates more than one cancer in the same quadrant of the breast, while *multicentric* means there is disease throughout the breast. Although LCIS does not metastasize, mastectomy was traditionally prescribed because the disease was often present in more than one place in the breast. However, LCIS can be bilateral in 30 to 50 percent of patients, so this often meant having a mastectomy on the affected side with a mirror-image biopsy of the other breast. If the biopsy was negative, then the patient was simply watched carefully. If positive, a bilateral mastectomy was done. Interestingly, if the LCIS had originally gone undetected twenty years ago and now you found an invasive lump, your treatment option would probably be lumpectomy and radiation, rather than the mastectomy the earlier stage then seemed to require.

Now we treat LCIS with lumpectomy and close follow-up. Studies have shown that up to 30 percent will develop an invasive breast cancer and that it can be in either breast and can take fifteen to twenty years to develop. Since the subsequent cancer can appear in either breast, the other treatment option is bilateral mastectomy and reconstruction.

Because more women nowadays get screening mammograms, the detection of early breast cancer, primarily ductal carcinoma in situ (DCIS), has increased. About 20 to 30 percent of breast cancers picked up by mammogram are DCIS. Treatment options are lumpectomy alone or with radiation, or mastectomy. Since radiation has been used for the early stage of invasive cancers it was felt that it should be tried with the DCIS also. But remember, DCIS rarely spreads to lymph nodes, so you may not need a lymph node dissection (discussed later in this chapter) as part of your treatment.

The treatment of DCIS is extremely controversial. In the past it was treated just like invasive breast cancer, with mastectomy, with almost 100 percent survival rate. Because 20 to 40 percent of these cancers are multicentric, or have small areas of invasive disease, some surgeons continue to recommend mastectomy, usually without a lymph node dissection. However, lumpectomy with radiation is a viable alternative to mastectomy if the area of DCIS is localized and can be completely removed with clear margins. If the cancer recurs, then mastectomy is needed.

The National Surgical Adjuvant Breast Project sponsored by the National Cancer Institute evaluated DCIS treated with lumpectomy alone versus DCIS treated with lumpectomy and radiation. This study was completed in 1992, and despite inaccuracies discovered in some Canadian data, results remain the same. LCIS is now under study. For information, call the NCI at 800-4-CANCER.

When Lumpectomy Is an Option

Most early breast cancers, Stage I and II, both invasive and noninvasive, qualify for lumpectomy if the tumor is 5 centimeters (2 inches) or less, and if your cancer is not multicentric or multifocal. Another consideration is the cosmetic result. A large tumor removed from a small breast can be disfiguring. Ideally, there should be no distortion of the breast by the lumpectomy and it should not involve the nipple-areola complex. So the size of the lump and your breast can sometimes determine treatment. You must also be willing to make the commitment to keeping your breast and following through with additional treatment such as radiation therapy.

Re-excision lumpectomy is simply "redoing" the biopsy and

removing the tissue that surrounded the tumor. At least a 1-centimeter margin of "grossly normal," cancer-free tissue is removed from the tumor bed. "Grossly" means what our eyes can see and what our fingers feel. This procedure leaves your breast intact, except for a small scar — the same scar as your biopsy. Lumpectomy may be the only treatment you need if your breast cancer is in situ. Otherwise, it may be followed by radiation if it is invasive. Chemotherapy may sometimes be added if there is a significant risk of systemic disease.

If your breast cancer recurs later in the same breast, then standard treatment would be mastectomy, because your breast could probably not tolerate radiation again. But re-excision and reradiation is now under study in Europe and by a few physicians in this country. If you did not have radiation with your first lumpectomy, then you could have another lumpectomy, this time with radiation. This may be possible with small, noninvasive tumors, but we have only begun to study this. We know that in localized early cancers, breast conservation and mastectomy are equally effective in both local control and survival.

Sometimes lumpectomy is called by other names, such as *partial mastectomy, re-excision, quadrantectomy, wedge resection.* Technically, it is a partial mastectomy in that part of the breast is removed. However, it is not a quadrantectomy or a wedge resection, which require removing as much as a quarter of the breast and truly are partial mastectomies. It is important to get clear with your surgeon on language. You want to know exactly what is happening. Are you getting a biopsy, a lumpectomy, or some form of mastectomy? Try to determine how much tissue will be removed.

When Lumpectomy Is Not an Option

Often, the size of the tumor would indicate that a lumpectomy is required, but if the follow-up therapy, such as radiation treatments, cannot be done, then mastectomy is the only course. Lumpectomy is not an option or not recommended in the following circumstances:

- If there is more than one cancerous lesion in your breast. Remember, multicentric cancer has multiple centers, or satellites, in different quadrants of your breast; multifocal lesions consist of two (or more) tiny growths in the same quadrant. (Occasionally, multifocal lesions are close enough to each other to be considered as one spot, and lumpectomy with radiation may be an option.)
- If you have a small breast and a large tumor. A large segment of tissue will need to be removed and could leave your breast disfigured.
- If you have a tumor right under your nipple. Again, removal of the tumor may be disfiguring.
- If you have collagen vascular disease, such as scleroderma. Your skin will be too sensitive to the radiation, and the cosmetic results will be poor. This is also true if you have lupus or vasculitis.
- If you have had radiation in the same breast or chest area, and cannot have it again. Mastectomy, with or without reconstruction, is recommended in this case.
- If you are not able or willing to commit to the many weeks of radiation treatment after a lumpectomy.
- If there is no facility in your area where you can obtain radiation treatment.
- If you would *prefer* a mastectomy — with or without reconstruction.

How to Know Which Type Mastectomy You Need

All the reasons that disqualify you for lumpectomy make you eligible for a mastectomy. There are several types of mastectomies — the simple mastectomy, the Patey modified radical, and the Halstead radical mastectomy. The difference between a modified radical and a radical is the amount of muscle removed with the breast.

A **simple mastectomy** removes the entire breast with the nipple-areola complex but no muscle or lymph nodes.

A **modified radical mastectomy** removes the entire breast with the nipple-areola complex, the lymph nodes, and the pectoralis minor chest muscle, but leaves the large pectoralis major intact behind your breast. In fact, if your tumor is stuck to the pectoralis, some surgeons may choose radiation over removing the pectoralis muscle. Other surgeons use a more traditional approach and remove the muscles if the tumor has extended into the muscle (radical mastectomy). The modified radical is the most commonly used mastectomy.

A **radical mastectomy** removes the breast, nipple-areola complex, the major and minor pectoralis muscles, and all the lymph nodes from the axilla (underarm) to the collarbone. In other words, all of your chest wall muscle is removed and your skin lies directly over your rib cage. A skin graft is sometimes taken from another area to sew onto your chest like a patch if your skin will not cover the incision and you have not elected to have reconstruction. Part of your axilla and the area around your collarbone is slightly hollowed out. Without your pectoralis muscle, your arm is less strong. And with more lymph nodes removed, your risk for infection or cellulitis in that arm is increased. Cellulitis is an infection of the soft tissue that can develop because your lymphatic system is less effective. Radical mastectomy is less common today and is used mostly for large tumors or lesions involving the chest wall muscles.

Why Some Lymph Nodes Are Removed

If you have invasive breast cancer, some of the lymph nodes under your arm are usually removed at the time of your lumpectomy or mastectomy to find out if any cancer has spread to the lymph system, the first place it would normally go. Lymph node status is one of the most important prognostic indicators, along with tumor size.

Lymph nodes are glands that act as the filters in your body's drainage system, and they are encased in fatty tissue in strategic locations throughout your body. We each have different sizes, shapes, and patterns of lymph nodes. Some people have heavy clusters of nodes, like bunches of grapes. Others have nodes spread out and far apart, like marbles dropped on the floor. Some nodes are as small as sesame seeds, others as big as jelly beans. Sometimes they are enlarged from infection or inflammation, or if they are filled with cancer cells. If your breast cancer is microinvasive or invasive there is potential for systemic spread. The lymph nodes are the best indicator of that risk. We look at three areas around the breast carefully.

- Supraclavicular, infraclavicular, and cervical nodes (the nodes around your collarbone and neck) are examined manually. When doctors feel your neck they are looking for enlarged lymph nodes. If the cancer has spread here, it is assumed to be systemic.

- Internal mammary lymph nodes cluster along the sides of the breastbone (sternum). If an invasive tumor is located in the upper inner quadrant of the breast, a CAT scan might be recommended to see behind the breastbone to try to determine if there are any enlarged lymph nodes, which would suggest tumor spread. This could help in determining a treatment plan. Few physicians prescribe this routinely, however.

- Axillary nodes are located under your arm, and tumors in the outer breast quadrant would send cancer cells to this location. The underarm nodes are easy to get to surgically and they provide the most information with the least disability.

It is sometimes possible to feel lymph nodes if they have tumor involvement, because they are usually swollen. If your doctor cannot find enlarged lymph nodes during a physical examination, then the odds are in your favor. Seventy percent of patients will not have metastasis to the nodes. Still, the best thing to do is take some out and look at them under the microscope. Almost everyone with invasive cancer, even very small tumors, has these lymph nodes checked.

It's possible to have a large tumor and no affected nodes. And it's possible to avoid mastectomy even with positive nodes. Each case must be treated individually. Metastasis to the lymph nodes does not necessarily mean there is an increased local recurrence rate. It does mean there's an increased risk for systemic recurrence. Radiation to your breast and axilla is a possible local treatment, while chemotherapy would be added as systemic treatment.

If you have "negative nodes" it means no cancer was found. "Positive nodes" means it has spread to the lymph nodes. "Micrometastasis" means less than 2 millimeters of metastasis is found in the node. "Extracapsular extension" means the tumor extends beyond the capsule, or wall, of the node and into the surrounding fat or soft tissue.

If cancer is found in the lymph nodes, you most likely need chemotherapy. If cancer has spread beyond the lymph nodes into the fatty tissue around them, you might need chemotherapy as systemic treatment, and local treatment with radiation to the area where the tumor has extended. If none of your lymph nodes show signs of cancer, you may still *elect* to have some kind of chemotherapy if you have invasive high-risk cancer. This decision would be based on the other prognostic factors, such as vascular or lymphatic involvement or the aggressiveness of your cancer cells. For more information about chemotherapy, see Chapter 8.

However, with more than four lymph nodes showing cancer, the risk of systemic and local recurrence increases, and therefore you should seek a consultation with both a medical and a radiation oncologist. Sometimes radiation will be added to the treatment plan, even with mastectomy, and it's important for you to meet with a radiation oncologist so you can understand all your options. If six to ten nodes are affected, more aggressive treatment, like bone marrow transplantation, is an option. Here again, go talk with a medical oncologist to find out what's involved. Bone marrow transplantation is still controversial but is used more and more often for breast cancer. There's a full explanation of this treatment in Chapter 9.

Getting Ready for Surgery

If you are having only a lumpectomy with no lymph node dissection, then surgery can be done on an outpatient basis. This will be done just like your biopsy (see Chapter 3). If you are having a lumpectomy with lymph node dissection, or a mastectomy and lymph node dissection, surgery is more complex and general anesthesia is used.

The risks of general anesthesia have decreased dramatically in recent years as drugs and technique have improved. However, ask the anesthesiologist what drugs will be used, and be forthcoming about *any* drugs or medications you are taking. For example, aspirin affects platelet function and can be associated with increased bruising. You may want to discuss with your doctor whether or not your menstrual cycle will have any effect on the surgery. Some feel midcycle is the best time for surgery, but there is still no hard data on this.

You are sedated before you enter the operating room, which may feel a bit chilly. The nurses and anesthesiologist get you ready. Your breast and arm are painted with antiseptic, and the rest of your body is covered with sterile drapes. Pneumatic boots may be put on your legs to help keep good circulation in your legs while you are asleep and to minimize the chance of a blood clot developing in your legs. During this time, while you are beginning to relax, your surgeon may come in and talk with you, so that you are feeling reassured as you drift off to sleep.

If You Are Having a Lumpectomy

Talk with your surgeon ahead of time about what kind of scar you will have. The re-excision lumpectomy generally follows the same incision as the biopsy. Curvilinear and circumareolar incisions follow the natural curve of your breast, your skin folds, or wrinkles. These incisions heal better than the straight or radial incisions used in the past, which were less sensitive to the appearance of the breast after surgery.

Lumpectomy is very similar to the biopsy, although slightly more tissue is taken out. Additional biopsy tissue may be taken from different sites inside the wound to check the margins. Often small metallic (titanium) clips are placed within the breast tissue at the corners of the wound to serve as markers for the radiation oncologist and for the radiologist for future mammograms. These are not removed. Your surgeon will probably operate with an electrocautery, a sort of electric scalpel that cuts and stops bleeding at the same time. A temporary drain may be put in place, and then the incision is sutured and dressed. The entire procedure usually takes twenty to forty minutes. If you are having an axillary dissection at the same time, it will take a bit longer. (See description below.)

If You Are Having a Mastectomy

Mastectomy and lymph node dissection takes one and a half to two and a half hours if no breast reconstruction is done at the same time. You and your surgeon are usually joined by the anesthesiologist, a nurse, and a resident or assistant. Generally, the incision is made in a horizontal direction, in the shape of an ellipse or oval around the nipple and biopsy scar. The breast is dissected away from the skin, which is peeled back. All the breast tissue between your collarbone and ribs and between your side and your center breastbone is removed. The breast is peeled away from the chest wall muscle (pectoralis), and then the lymph nodes are dissected out — unless you are having a simple mastectomy, when no nodes are removed. With a modified radical or radical mastectomy, some of your chest muscle is removed, too. The area is checked to be certain there is no bleeding and then drained and sutured closed. Dressings are placed.

Until the mid-1980s, mastectomy kept women hospitalized for two weeks or more until they healed well enough for stitches and drains to be removed. Now we know it is much better to recover at home, so a hospital stay is from one to three days. Another day or more may be added if you have immediate reconstruction. Reconstruction is something to think about *before* mastectomy. We encourage our mastectomy patients to see plastic surgeons even if they don't think they want reconstruction. They may change their minds later and we want them to know what their options are. Try to think through each alternative and decide which is the best for you and your lifestyle. In the next chapter you will find information on various types of reconstruction.

If You Are Having an Axillary (Lymph Node) Dissection

A simple 2-to-3-inch curved incision in the skin crease under the arm allows us access to the lymph nodes. (The longer radial incision from the underarm to the breast, once common practice, is no longer used.) If you have a modified radical mastectomy, all of your axillary nodes will be removed; with lumpectomy, some will be removed; and with simple mastectomy, none.

There is no prescribed number of lymph nodes to look at, but at least ten should be removed. Each node removed is examined carefully by the pathologist. However, even if the nodes are negative (no tumor seen), some women with invasive breast cancer will develop metastatic disease. Once the surgeon removes the tissue containing the lymph nodes, the pathologist presses through the fatty tissue to free all of the lymph nodes for inspection. In a small hospital with a standard pathology staff, only ten or fifteen nodes may be identified. At a larger medical center, where residents assist pathologists, twenty to thirty nodes may be identified. Results depend on

the amount of tissue removed from your axilla and the dili-
gence of the pathologist.

How Will Axillary Dissection Affect My Arm?

Having lymph nodes removed from your underarm after surgery has some permanent effect on you, but with care, you will
hardly notice. Sometimes, if the intercostal nerve is stretched
out or if it is cut, you may be numb in the upper arm and
underarm. This is the sensory nerve that crosses through the
axilla to supply sensation along the inside of your arm, from
your underarm to your elbow. For two to four weeks you might
feel numbness, then pins and needles or burning feelings for
a couple of weeks. It usually takes about a year to get all the
feeling back. The range-of-motion and flexibility exercises
described in Chapter 14 take only a few minutes out of each
day. But if you do them regularly, your arm will get back into
shape quickly. If you have subtle movement problems, or want
more support or muscle strength, physical therapy can help.

Up to 10 percent of women get lymphedema, swelling of
the arm. Because you have fewer lymph nodes (and the lymphatic channels have been disrupted by surgery) to act as
catch basins in that area, your arm can more easily become
infected, resulting in swelling. Lymphedema is usually progres-
sive, and it can be a chronic problem even without infection.
You may be fine for years and one day a paper cut may cause
your arm to swell. However, if treated early, it may be controlled or reversed. Chapter 14 discusses how to prevent and
treat lymphedema.

Waking Up in the Recovery Room

Whether you had a lumpectomy and axillary dissection or a
mastectomy, when you wake up, you will find a bulky dressing
on your breast, held in place with swaddling around your chest
like an elastic bandage. Your arm may be in a sling, or tem-

porarily held against your side with the swaddling. One or two drains are attached to your incisions, and you empty these twice a day for ten to fourteen days. Eventually, your body takes over and the drainage will decrease so drains can be removed.

If you had lumpectomy and lymph node dissection, you probably have only one drain, and most of your discomfort — if any — is under your arm. With mastectomy and lymph node dissection, you have as many as two drains to handle. (More drains may be in place in the abdomen if reconstruction is performed at the same time.) Your chest wall feels numb.

Most women are able to tolerate food twelve hours after surgery, and until then you are fed intravenously. A nurse checks your vital signs periodically and rubs your feet and hands to keep blood circulating. You may wear the pneumatic boots until you get out of bed to walk around — and you are encouraged to do that as soon as you can.

The Day After Surgery

Once you have fully recovered from the effects of anesthesia, you are encouraged to eat, walk around, and start moving your arm. You may be groggy, or you may feel energized. People react differently to surgery and anesthesia. Your chest will be numb after a mastectomy, especially around the incision. When the numbness wears off, a tight feeling develops.

Ask your surgeon to be with you when the dressing is removed for the first time. This is an emotionally traumatic time. Some women want to be absolutely alone when they see the wound where their breast once was. Others want only their husbands or lovers around. You should be able to do this however you want, but it is easier to have your doctor or an experienced nurse help you.

One woman who had a mastectomy in a small suburban hospital told us nobody came to help her remove the dressing the day after surgery. Finally, a young, inexperienced female nurse, who had never seen a mastectomy, came in to change the dressing. The nurse was so shaken that the patient had to console her. This is not the way it should be, so find out in advance what the procedure will be.

Ask to see a Reach to Recovery volunteer if you like. These breast cancer survivors have been trained by the American Cancer Society to help others cope right after surgery. They often bring a prosthesis with them, or talk with you about reconstruction. These women also have insight into what you are feeling, and can listen and discuss your concerns and give you direction about physical therapy or support groups. Keep in mind that you always have the option of having delayed reconstruction at any time in the future.

Before you leave the hospital be sure to get written instructions about how to care for your incisions and drains at home. Instructions for home care should include what pain medications to take if you need them, signs of infection to watch for, problems with drains, when to take a shower, when to see the doctor, how often to change your dressing, whether or not to wear a bra, when to start exercising, and any limitations on lifting (such as to avoid lifting anything weighing more than twenty-five pounds).

Recovering at Home

At home wear a snug cotton undershirt, tank top, or one of the long soft bras — crop tops — now available. These are comfortable, will breathe with you, and hold your dressing in place. (They wash easily, too.) Stuff some extra bandages underneath for symmetry with your other side. Buy these ahead of time, so you have them when you get home.

Drains. A thin tube of clear plastic allows the drainage of blood and serous fluid into a bubble-type reservoir you can pin to your undershirt. Initially, the fluid will be bloody; it will gradually become yellow. About 50–200 cubic centimeters (cc) of fluid — an ounce is 30 cc — a day will collect in the reservoir, which is calibrated so you can keep track of the amount of fluid. Empty the drain twice a day, and ask your doctor if you should record the amount. This will let you know if it is diminishing as it should. There is a port on the bottom part of the bulb which unplugs, so you can empty it easily.

Incisions. Don't get your incision wet for one day. After that, showers are okay. Pat yourself dry and reapply your dressings. Check your wound for any signs of infection, such as redness, swelling, or oozing. Pin your drains onto your wrap or T-shirt.

After mastectomy, you may experience numbness or tingling around your chest wall scar if a nerve was cut. This happens often. You may also experience feelings in your missing breast, the phantom pain often experienced by people who lose an arm or leg. Your brain's signals are not yet adjusted to the new situation. If you develop a seroma, which is like a big blister of fluid collected under the skin, your surgeon needs to drain (aspirate) this every week. Seromas are quite common and not a cause for worry.

Exercise. The best way to restore the power to your arm is to start exercising it a day or two after surgery. Ask your doctor and nurses, or the hospital physical therapist, to help you begin before you leave the hospital. Here are some exercises you can do while lying in bed. Always breathe deeply and evenly so you are calm and relaxed when you begin exercising. Sometimes you will be more relaxed after a shower, and you may choose to do the exercises at this time, so they are more effective. Do these three times a day and repeat each exercise at least ten times.

- While lying on your back in bed, raise your arm straight up and back to touch the headboard.
- Rotate your shoulders forward, then down and back in circles to loosen your upper back and chest muscles.
- Clasp your hands behind your head and push your elbows into the mattress.

- With your arm raised, clench and unclench your fist, or squeeze a rubber ball.

  Once you are up and around, do range-of-motion exercises (see page 166) to retrain your muscles to your altered body.

Your spirit. A period of depression strikes everyone at some time during breast cancer treatment. You've had a real loss, and grief is part of getting through it. You may be depressed right after mastectomy, but things improve after this. With a lumpectomy and radiation, the depression sometimes begins after the weeks of radiation are over. Up until then you've had the daily treatments to distract you. Now you feel isolated and this is when you need the company of other women who know the feelings. Go visit your support group! You need them now.

Follow-up care for breast cancer surgery is like that for any surgery. Eat well, sleep well, watch out for infection, and resume your normal routine as soon as possible. Visit your surgeon a week or two after surgery for suture removal and to check on the healing process. If you had reconstruction, then you have more people to see. Drains are usually removed at these early visits. Visit the radiation therapist and chemotherapist if that's on your agenda. It is standard to see a chemotherapist for a consultation even with negative nodes, as more and more women are offered adjuvant chemotherapy or hormone therapy to minimize any risk.

During the next two years you will be examined about every three months. After that it will be less often, but for the rest of your life, regularly scheduled checkups are mandatory! There is more detail about follow-up care in the next section of the book.

✔ Questions to Ask Before Surgery

These questions are meant to help you interview physicians and other healthcare professionals so that you can feel secure about your treatment decisions. Some of these questions have no clear-cut answers, some do. But ask anyway!

Describe the breast procedure and the extent of the axillary dissection.

To avoid any surprises after surgery, find out what to expect, how you will feel and look when you see your body after surgery. The surgeon should explain where and how big all incisions will be, how surgery will affect your physical movement, how long recovery will take. Often you will be shown photographs to give you a clear idea of what to expect.

What are the risks and side effects of this surgery?

There is always a risk with anesthesia, but it is extremely low, especially if you are in good health. Immediate side effects could be pain or swelling. Bleeding and infection could occur but rarely do. Long-term effects could be lymphedema, numbness, or loss of some movement in your arm.

What will happen if I do not have this procedure?

To understand your need for surgery, it is helpful to understand what will happen if you do not have it. Ask about the risk for subsequent local or distant recurrence.

How many lymph nodes will you remove?

With a lumpectomy, expect fifteen to twenty nodes. With a mastectomy, twenty to twenty-five nodes. In larger hospitals, with larger pathology staffs, even more nodes may be identified in the tissue specimen for inspection.

When will you have the pathology report on my lymph node status?

Your doctor should know within seventy-two hours, but the official typed report takes about two weeks to arrive. Most physicians will tell you about this report at your next visit. However, if you are anxious, call and ask.

Will my surgeon be with me the first time the dressing is changed?

Most surgeons will want to see your incision and change your dressing. This may not be standard everywhere, however. Another physician or a nurse may do this.

Will I receive written instructions for care for my incisions and drains?

Hospitals are getting better about patient education, and most will give you at least a sheet of paper with minimal instructions on follow-up care. But ask to make sure. Your local American Cancer Society chapter has this information, too.

How often will I see my surgeon afterward?

After immediate follow-up, removing drains and sutures, you should see your surgeon every three or four months for the first two years to monitor progress of your healing as well as to check for signs of recurrence.

Do you accept my medical insurance for all the charges involved?

Always find out what your insurance covers. There are many charges connected with surgery, such as the use of the operating room, anesthesia, use of the recovery room, medications, sometimes bandages, cost of the hospital room, and meals. Remember to check your policy for the second-opinion requirement. Some won't pay for surgery unless you have gotten a second opinion — in writing.

~ 6

After Mastectomy:
Reconstruction or Prosthesis?

Many short- and long-term considerations are involved in your decision to have breast reconstruction or wear a prosthesis. What will your reconstructed breast look like in ten years? Will it gain and lose weight with you? What can be done if you don't like it? What if your breast cancer recurs? We always refer mastectomy patients to a plastic surgeon — even if they say they do not want reconstruction. It's good to know about it anyway, to be informed about your options.

Your choices for reconstructive surgery may depend to some extent on how much muscle and lymph tissue was removed after mastectomy and how much tissue remains. The plastic surgeon's experience with each technique and your own preferences are also major considerations.

Think about your other breast, too. Will it need to be adjusted to match the new one? If you are full breasted, a matching reconstructed breast may not turn out as well as you'd like. Conversely, if you have very small breasts, you may want to have bigger breasts. Now's your chance! Some women have elected to have a prophylactic mastectomy on the opposite side in order to have two matching reconstructed breasts, but this is the exception. (Women from families with a history of breast cancer often have prophylactic mastectomy, too.)

Ask yourself how you feel about your surviving breast before you alter it. Two new breasts may be more than you want to cope with. Work with your plastic surgeon to identify your needs and concerns, and approach reconstruction with realistic expectations.

If reconstruction begins when you have your mastectomy, you avoid the flat postoperative look. It was once thought that women needed to experience that flatness in order to appreciate reconstruction. We have learned that isn't necessarily so. Past reconstructions used implants that often were hard, immobile, and artificial looking. Today, implants are adjustable and more natural looking. When your breasts are reconstructed with your own tissue and skin, they look and feel soft and natural.

Women of all ages have reconstruction, and some who had mastectomies twenty years ago have recently decided to have reconstruction. Past attitudes about age often assumed mature women did not care about their breasts anymore, so reconstruction was rarely offered to them. The same bias has been true of women with limited financial resources. It was assumed they could not afford it. But reconstruction is *not* cosmetic surgery — it is part of your breast cancer treatment, and is now covered by health insurance, including Medicare.

It may not be wise to have reconstructive surgery if you smoke or if you have diabetes or heart or lung disease. Healing can be difficult or delayed, but each case must be evaluated individually. If you cannot commit to the long and sometimes tedious follow-up treatments and procedures necessary for a successful reconstruction, then a prosthesis might be best for you.

The most important considerations for reconstructive surgery are that you are in good health and that you want very much to take it on. Once that's decided, you can choose from several forms of reconstruction. The decision between an implant and reconstruction with your own tissue is an important one. Know also that it takes a highly skilled plastic surgeon with vast experience in breast reconstruction to do this job well. So get all the information you want before you decide.

If you are going to need chemotherapy, you will not be able

to have reconstruction until two or three months after chemotherapy ends unless you have reconstruction at the same time as the mastectomy and before you start chemotherapy. The second stage of reconstruction (nipple reconstruction or modeling and shaping) is delayed until after chemotherapy ends. The disadvantage of immediate reconstruction is that the total operation is longer and more complicated than a mastectomy alone. There may be some additional blood loss and potential wound-healing problems.

A simple saline implant or tissue-expander implant under existing skin is the simplest breast reconstruction. The expander is an adjustable implant that gradually forces your skin to expand to the necessary size. Complexity increases for reconstruction with a flap of your own tissue — a piece of skin, muscle, and fat, transferred from another part of your body to your chest wall — to fashion a complete breast. Certain flap reconstructions can add as much as six to eight hours to the operating time following mastectomy and are the most complex reconstructions.

Don't let possibilities overwhelm you. Think about the advantages and disadvantages of each type of reconstruction. Write them down. Talk with women who have had reconstruction. Ask them to show you their breasts and the donor sites. Talk with a Reach to Recovery volunteer who has had reconstructive breast surgery. Then go for the simplest and safest procedure that you will feel good about.

Reconstruction with Implants

Implant reconstruction is suitable if your breasts are small or firm. If your breasts are large, you may not have enough tissue available after your mastectomy to stretch around an implant of matching size — unless you plan a reduction of the other breast. Implants are not suitable if you don't have enough muscle and skin left on your chest, you have had previous radiation to your breast, or you simply do not want a foreign object in your body.

Saline-filled implants have been in use since the 1960s, and most women have never had them removed or replaced. A saline implant is a round silicone envelope filled with salt water. The risk of leakage is about 2 percent, but because this is salt water, it does no harm. Your body simply absorbs it.

Silicone-filled implants. These implants are unavailable until the Federal Drug Administration completes a study on their safety. They were removed from the market when some of them leaked and caused toxic reactions. Silicone gel implants were thought to feel the most natural, and many women still have these implants without problem.

Tissue expanders are adjustable implants that can be inflated after they are placed. Your skin stretches out the way it does when you are pregnant. Once your breast is removed and checked by the pathologist, the plastic surgeon positions the expander under the layer of chest muscle and the muscle layer is sutured. A narrow tube with a valve projects from the implant and out under the skin under your arm. The implant is gradually inflated — over a period of weeks or months — with saline. Then a smaller implant replaces the expander and the loosened skin is used to create a more natural fold under your breast. Tissue expanders are suitable after a simple or modified radical mastectomy if your chest muscles are intact. There is, naturally, a limit as to how much your skin can expand, which is why these are less suitable if you have full breasts.

When Implant Reconstruction Follows Mastectomy

The implant procedure can sometimes be done on an outpatient basis if you do not have it at the same time as your mastectomy. It takes an hour or two with general anesthesia. Occasionally it is done with intravenous sedation. Your mastectomy scar is reopened and the implant inserted behind your chest muscle. Implants are placed behind the chest muscle for a smoother and firmer contour and so that they don't harden.

However, it is a good idea to massage your new breast frequently to keep the implant soft. Review this with your plastic surgeon.

Although the implant is positioned for the best symmetry with your other breast, this is not always attainable in one procedure. A second procedure may be necessary to adjust the shape and projection, with possibly a third procedure to add the nipple.

After Your Implant Is Placed

After surgery — with the saline implant or the expander — your breast may look flat because your chest muscle is tight, but as the muscle stretches out over a period of months your breast will assume a more natural shape and projection. If your implant needs to be held in place or guided downward, a tube top or flat dressing is used after surgery. If it needs to be guided upward, you need to wear a bra all the time. The stitches either dissolve or are removed in a week. Recovery takes a day or two, and within a few weeks you can resume full activity with your arm and shoulder.

However, with a tissue expander, the process is still not complete. It takes many visits to your plastic surgeon to expand your implant. At each visit, which lasts fifteen to thirty minutes, saline is added to the expander through the valve under your arm. Your progress depends on how much expansion you can tolerate. In some cases each new expansion can hurt. Once the expansion is completed, another surgical procedure may be necessary to model and shape your breast and form the crease between the bottom of your breast and the chest wall.

What Complications Are Possible with Implants?

Fibrous *capsular contracture* is a thick scarring that forms around the implant because your body is trying to reject it. This may soften over time, or it can become more dense and tender.

Newer implants have a rough outer surface and don't seem to develop this reaction. There is some scar tissue around all implants, which is why most reconstructed breasts with implants feel firmer than normal. However, if the capsular contracture causes your breast to look deformed, then it must be surgically removed and replaced or covered with a tissue flap. Sometimes a flap is pulled around from your back to provide more tissue to cover the implant. Flaps from other areas can be used if necessary. Where the flap comes from is usually determined by the amount of tissue needed, the integrity of the muscles involved, and patient preference based on the side effects of each surgery and where the scars will be.

An implant can rupture, but usually only from severe trauma, as in an automobile accident. Saline implants can rupture more easily than silicone-filled implants, but the saline is not going to be toxic if it gets into your system. Your body absorbs the extra salt water, and the implant deflates and can be replaced. An implant can also deflate over a period of time, and this occurs in about 2 percent of cases. Another 1 or 2 percent of women will develop infections, which need to be treated promptly with antibiotics. Smokers are especially susceptible to infection.

Advantages and Disadvantages of Implant Reconstruction

The greatest advantages of implant reconstruction over tissue-flap reconstruction are that you avoid lengthy surgery, you recover right away, and it's much cheaper. You also avoid injuring your abdominal muscle (which can occur with TRAM-flap reconstruction, described below) and losing skin from other parts of your body. However, you do need to follow through with expansion treatments and the final nip-and-tuck procedure, if you want a satisfactory result.

Disadvantages are that your breast will not feel as soft and natural as one that is reconstructed with your own flesh, it

won't gain and lose weight with you, and it won't droop like
the other one. An implant is also a foreign object.

Does an Implant Interfere with Breast Cancer Therapy?

No. If reconstruction is done immediately after mastectomy,
there is rarely a delay in starting adjuvant chemotherapy. A
delayed implant procedure can be done two or three months
after chemotherapy ends. Then, once your white blood count
has been restored, your risk of infection will be diminished.

Reconstruction can generally be done six weeks after radiation therapy to the chest wall.

What Should I Know About My Implant?

A breast implant comes in a package just like any pharmaceutical product. Keep the instructions from the package with
your medical records. Record the date, manufacturer's name,
and other pertinent information. There are several resources
for information about breast implants.

- **Breast Implant Information Line**   800-532-4440
  U.S. Food and Drug Administration will send you an information packet.

- **International Breast Implant Registry**   800-892-9211
  Breast implants are part of the Medic Alert system. If you
  register, you get a bracelet that identifies you as wearing an
  implant.

- **NABCO Hotline**   212-719-0154
  Ask for current information sheets on breast implants.

Reconstruction with Your Own Tissue Flap

There is a big difference between implant reconstruction and more complicated breast reconstruction with your own tissue, which involves longer and more complex surgery, and has more potential complications. Recovery takes longer, and additional surgical procedures may be needed before you have the best possible breast.

A complete breast is fashioned with flaps of tissue from the transverse rectus abdominus muscle (abdomen), the latissimus dorsi muscle (back), or the gluteus maximus muscle (buttock). Breast reconstruction with your own flesh is a good way to get the most natural-looking breast and one that most closely resembles your other breast. It will change with your body because it *is* your body. It will gain and lose weight with you. It will feel soft and smooth (eventually) and even jiggle like a normal breast. It will look better than an implant, particularly if you have had radical mastectomy with more deformity, or if previous radiation left you with thicker skin. There is the added bonus of taking away some flesh where you may not need it — tummy or buttocks — and leaving you slimmer. There are two kinds of flaps used in reconstruction:

- A *pedicle flap* remains attached at one end to the original (donor) tissue and blood supply in the back or abdomen and is rotated around or pulled up to the chest wall site.

- A *free flap* is completely detached from its original site (generally the abdomen or buttock) and is nourished by a set of blood vessels (one artery and one vein) which are sewn — using microsurgery — into the vessels in the axilla to keep the flap alive. Because of the length of time for the operation, the free flap can lose blood and die before it is relocated and connected to its new blood supply. Blood vessels can also clot or go into spasm and limit blood flow.

Most common reconstructions are done with pedicle flaps from the abdomen or back, and free flaps from the abdomen or buttock.

When You Should Not Have Flap Reconstruction

No pedicle or free-tissue-flap reconstruction can be done if you smoke, because of the importance of the isolated and limited blood supply to the flap. When you smoke, your blood vessels become constricted and can go into spasm from the nicotine; such vessels won't allow the flap to get enough blood to stay alive during surgery. If the flap dies, it cannot be used. This means the surgery will have to be done again at a later time.

Because reconstruction is major surgery and involves prolonged anesthesia and an extended healing period, be sure your emotions and personal circumstances are such that you can cope with it. If you have any chronic health conditions such as diabetes or a heart or lung disorder, give this careful thought and discuss it with all of your doctors. Remember, you can always change your mind and have reconstruction done some other time.

What Is a TRAM Reconstruction?

The TRAM flap is the most common of the reconstructions. The surgery takes from three to six hours. If you are having it done immediately following mastectomy, you could be in the operating room for as long as eight or nine hours in all. Most surgeons have you donate your own blood ahead of time in case you need it during surgery. This reconstruction uses a long strip of skin, muscle, and fatty tissue — about 4 by 8 inches — from your abdomen to build a breast.

Your plastic surgeon designs a flap (with a felt-tip pen) along your mid- to lower abdomen. An incision is made from hip to hip. The TRAM (transverse rectus abdominus muscle) is cut at the bottom and then tunneled up over your ribs and under your skin. The top of the flap is sewn in place at the clavicle and the lower portion folded and contoured and checked for symmetry with your other breast. You are pulled into a sitting position to make sure the new breast is symmetrical with the other. Then it is sewn into place. On your breast you will have an elliptic stitch pattern from the lower breast crease and up toward the nipple. You will have a transverse scar across your lower abdomen, like that of a tummy tuck (a common procedure done to slim the abdomen).

The TRAM-flap procedure was developed in the early 1980s and is now the most-used flap procedure and has the best results. A TRAM can only be done once, however. If future reconstruction is needed on your breast, it must be done some other way.

Because your tissue flap is moving a long distance from your lower abdomen up to your breast, the flap needs a good blood supply. You must be healthy for this procedure to be successful. It cannot be done if you smoke, because your blood vessels are too constricted. Even if you are a former smoker, your blood vessels may already be too damaged to handle this procedure. If you are overweight, or have had liposuction in the past, you would not be able to have a TRAM reconstruction. Very thin women may also be disqualified if they don't have enough flesh on the abdomen. Women with diabetes, heart disease, or who have had a stroke are poor risks for this surgery.

In the past, it was not possible to do TRAM flap if you wanted to become pregnant later, because too much skin and muscle was taken from the abdomen. Now we have learned how to do it so that the abdomen muscle is split, and this allows the abdomen wall to stretch out as the fetus matures. If the abdomen muscles stretch apart too much, they can be repaired after childbirth.

Recovering from a TRAM Reconstruction

You feel like you've been in a train wreck for the first two days after a TRAM flap. It's similar to the feeling after a C-section or a tummy tuck. You cannot stand up straight, and you have to walk around dragging a rack with an intravenous bag and a Foley catheter. You won't be able to do sit-ups for quite a while, but this will all pass.

You may avoid some of the post-op anemia that will leave you weak, tearful, and feeling run-down by getting a blood transfusion. (If you donate your own blood ahead of time, you can avoid the risk of infection.) Your body has been through an enormous ordeal. Relax and give yourself time to recover. Many women today feel so pressured to do everything, they don't give themselves any downtime to recuperate. Let everything else go.

Your hospital bed is flexed so there is no tension on your abdomen, and to keep blood flowing in your legs. You need to get up and walk the next day. This is important to keep the blood flowing. You may find two drains in your breast and three or four attached to your abdomen. These can remain for as long as two weeks. You receive standard postoperative care for the first twenty-four hours, and then the dressings are removed and your incisions are covered with light dressings until they heal.

Despite the battered appearance of their new breast, most women respond well to their first look at it. Initially, a flap-built breast is swollen and bruised. It looks like it was beaten up, and it was. Your breast may feel cool and hard until good blood flow is established. It softens over time.

You will be discharged from the hospital in four or five days. You may need pain medications for a few days after you go home. Within six or eight weeks you'll be back to normal. Exercise to strengthen your abdomen may be advised later by your doctor. Some women have to push themselves up from a reclining position for a while.

What Complications Are Possible with a TRAM Flap?

While your new breast settles in, the fat sometimes hardens during healing and forms little lumps that feel like tumors. This can be checked by your doctor. The lumps should soften in six to eight weeks. Occasionally this hardened fat (fat necrosis) is surgically removed as an outpatient procedure. Sometimes healing takes longer if the blood supply to the new flap is insufficient. Fluid can collect in the breast and form a seroma. This has to be aspirated in your doctor's office. As with any surgery, there are slight risks of bleeding, hematoma, infection, or blood clots in the legs. The additional risk of this surgery is abdominal hernia.

The Latissimus Dorsi Flap

Reconstruction with the latissimus dorsi muscle can be done to supplement an implant or by itself, if your breasts are not too large. With this procedure during mastectomy, the latissimus flap can be pulled around from your back. This reconstruction takes less time than the TRAM (two to four hours) and has a shorter recovery period. You have a single oblique scar in the middle of your back, generally hidden under the bra line, or a diagonal scar under your arm. You may always have a slight bulge under your arm where the skin, muscle, and fat was tunneled through, and be a bit lopsided because your back is thinner on one side.

Recovering from a Latissimus Dorsi Flap

You have drains in front and back, and you need to limit arm and shoulder activity for a few days. The exercise causes fluid to collect in the surgical area and this increases drainage. Fluid can collect in your back, and a drain may have to be reinserted or the fluid aspirated.

You'll be in the hospital three to six days. Pain or soreness in your back and underarm subsides in two to three weeks as your arm regains normal activity. The loss of this muscle in your back may cause your shoulder to move forward, but exercise can retrain your other muscles to compensate for this.

Free-Flap Reconstruction with Gluteus Maximus

Reconstruction with a free flap from your buttock is the most demanding and complex of the procedures, so you need an expert who does hundreds of procedures, because many things can go wrong. Check the surgeon's success rate by asking how many of these reconstructions he or she has done. If the answer seems too minimal (very few surgeons have experience with this procedure on a regular basis), try someone else. This technique is generally used if your TRAM muscle is insufficient. A microsurgeon works with your breast surgeon and your plastic surgeon, so there is quite a crowd in the operating room.

You must be psyched for this operation. It can mean eight hours or more under anesthesia. Success depends on the microsurgery techniques, and the plastic surgeon's design. A flap is cut from the middle or bottom of your buttock. The lower part is preferred because the scar will be hidden, and the blood vessels are larger there. Once the flap is cut, it is immediately reattached by the feeder blood vessel to the vessels under your arm. This is done under the microscope. Your buttock is sutured and the flap is sewn to your chest wall and shaped, the same way as the other flaps.

This surgery depends on a single set of blood vessels, which could possibly be traumatized by a clot or go into spasm. Blood-flow failure to the flap would mean having to reoperate. The back of your thigh could be numb if your nerve is divided during the procedure.

Recovering from a Gluteal Free Flap

This recovery is not as painful as recovering from the TRAM, but you will have to lie on your side for several days and sit on a "donut" until you are able to withstand normal pressure on your buttock. You remain hospitalized for six to eight days, with drains in your breast and buttock for three or four days.

Sometimes drains have to go home with you until production of fluid subsides. You may have to restrict movement in your arm and shoulder for a few days, and take antibiotics for the first four days or more. In six to eight weeks you should be able to resume normal activity.

Follow-up Procedures

You are not finished yet. For best results, you probably will need a second procedure months later to refine the contour of the new breast. This can include removing excess tissue or scars or fat necrosis. If a permanent implant is needed to replace the expander, it is done then. Expanders are almost always used with implants now because the results are so much better if the skin is overstretched before placing the permanent implant. The nipple may be added at this time, or later if too much else is going on.

How Is a Nipple Reconstructed?

Building a new nipple is a second operation, after your new breast has had a chance to settle into its new shape and your scars have healed — after three to six months. This is often done as an outpatient procedure. In the past, skin was grafted from the inner thigh or the back of the ear because the coloring best matched the nipple. Now skin is most often taken from the same breast and shaped into a nipple. Occasionally, skin is taken from the opposite areola. This results in both areolas being smaller, but the alteration is minimal. The color match for the nipple and areola is achieved with tattooing. Keep in mind, this is not a real nipple and it will have no feeling or function other than a cosmetic one.

Getting Used to Your New Breast

Don't expect your new breast to look exactly like the one you lost. For the first few weeks it won't look very attractive. It's a good idea to prepare yourself so that your expectations mesh with postoperative realities. Although you understood intellectually ahead of time, emotionally you still must cope with the reality of scars, bruises, redness, and pain in donor areas. It's a difficult confrontation, but most women are just glad that reconstruction has begun.

Your new breast will ultimately feel soft, mushy — like a breast. It jiggles once it is healed. It may never have the same projection your old breast did, but some feeling will return to your breast, depending upon how many nerves regenerate. Your nipple, however, will never have any feeling.

What About Doing Breast Self-exam?

It is imperative to continue doing BSE on your reconstructed breast as well as your other breast. Check the skin of your new breast religiously for rashes, nodules, masses, or any change.

Choosing a Plastic Surgeon

You really have to like your plastic surgeon. Reconstruction is an emotion-packed procedure, and you must be able to talk candidly about your *feelings* about your breasts. Bring your spouse or partner to this interview, too. Everybody's feelings should be aired now. How you feel about your plastic surgeon affects your response to surgery. Look at pictures of reconstructed breasts and donor sites — before and after, and long after — so you know what to expect about scars, bruising, healing, pain, and long-term effects. You want as few surprises as possible.

The plastic surgeon you choose must have extensive experience in breast reconstruction. Try to find out the types of reconstruction favored by the surgeon. All doctors have biases. Also interview the microsurgeon who may be part of the team for this surgery. Expect your plastic surgeon to work closely with your breast surgeon, and to consult with your other doctors, including the pathologist.

Your breast surgeon will probably refer you to a plastic surgeon, who may be part of the breast management team in your hospital. But you can also get referrals from other women, from your American Cancer Society chapter, especially the Reach to Recovery volunteers, and various organizational hotlines. You can also get a list of board-certified plastic reconstructive surgeons in your area by calling the American Society of Plastic and Reconstructive Surgeons referral line, 800-635-0635.

What Does Reconstruction Cost?

Depending on the procedure, the surgical fee for reconstructive breast surgery can range from $1,500 to as much as $10,000. Implant reconstruction is cheaper than flap reconstruction, but you must also pay for the implant itself, as well as the expansion sessions in the months following the implant procedure. Reconstructive surgery is less expensive if it is done immediately following mastectomy, because you are already in the operating room under anesthesia.

Find out all of the costs in advance so you can evaluate your options thoroughly. Because breast reconstruction is not cosmetic surgery, most medical insurance — including Medicare and Medicaid — covers part or all of the cost. Many states require insurance coverage for reconstructive surgery. Because insurance coverage varies, be certain that all followup procedures are included. Also find out if both breasts are covered if you choose to have prophylactic reconstruction on the other side. If you are not insured and have limited income, call the plastic surgery division in a university teaching hospital. Some offer breast reconstruction at reduced cost.

If You Choose an External Prosthesis

A month or six weeks after surgery you are healed enough to be fitted for a permanent prosthesis. Millions of women wear breast prostheses without a problem. Prostheses look more realistic than they used to. Still, it takes some shopping around and trying on several types to find one that feels comfortable and gives you symmetry with your other breast. Some lingerie shops specialize in fittings.

Prostheses come in a variety of styles. They can be covered with soft fabric or plastic, or encased in a silicone envelope. Some are simply foam rubber pads, and others are filled with water, air, chemical gel, or ceramic particles. They can be designed specifically for the right or left side, with or without a nipple. Some can be worn without a bra, and custom forms adhere directly to your chest wall and closely match your other breast. (These require individual molds to be made; the prosthesis is glued to the chest wall and makeup is often used to mask the edges.) Very small prostheses, called equalizers, fit women who have had a partial mastectomy. Extremely light-weight forms are available to wear in a nightgown or with sports clothes.

How to Select the Right Prosthesis

First, find a bra that fits well and will hold the form in place. This may be one of your favorite bras — as long as it is not underwired — or you may have to shop around. Special mastectomy bras are built up to cover a form and have wider straps and pockets inside the cup. A pocket can be sewn into your bathing suit and your standard bras to keep the form in place. A Reach to Recovery volunteer from the American Cancer Society can show you some of the different types.

Some specialty stores have professional fitters — some will even come to your home — and carry special lingerie and sports-wear as well. A properly fitting prosthesis feels comfortable and stays in place when you move. At first it may feel heavy, but you will get used to the extra weight. It's worth the shopping-around time to get one that feels right. If it is uncomfortable, it is a constant reminder that you have lost a breast. Find out if the form absorbs perspiration or other chemicals from your skin and how to clean and care for it. Take a close friend with you to help with your clothes and for moral support.

Prostheses cost anywhere from $10 to $400 and most are guaranteed for five years. Custom forms cost up to $1,000. Most medical insurance covers this expense, but you may be limited to a certain number of prostheses and bras, perhaps one per year. Get a written prescription for the prosthesis, bras, and bathing suits from your surgeon to guarantee payment. Most stores accept Medicare.

Ask your hospital social worker or your Reach to Recovery volunteer, or check the yellow pages under Lingerie, Brassieres, Breast Prostheses, or Surgical Supply. You can also call:

- **American Cancer Society**   800-ACS-2345
  Your local chapter may have a prosthesis bank, and the Reach to Recovery volunteer may also be a resource.
- **Y-ME National Hotline**   800-221-2142
  This group maintains a prosthesis bank for women with limited resources.

✔ Questions to Ask About Breast Reconstruction

These questions are meant to help you interview physicians and other healthcare professionals so that you can feel secure about your treatment decisions. Some of these questions have no clear-cut answers, some do. But ask anyway!

What types of breast reconstruction have you done?

A plastic surgeon must be experienced in breast reconstruction, but some may have biases toward certain types of implant or tissue reconstruction, such as the TRAM, latissimus dorsi, or gluteus maximus flap. A plastic surgeon may have done hundreds of TRAMs but only one gluteal free flap.

Should I have it done at the time of mastectomy, or later?

Immediate reconstruction saves you the costs and risks of another anesthesia and surgery later. Immediate reconstruction may be advisable if you are planning to have chemotherapy within a few weeks after surgery. Otherwise, you would have to wait eight to nine months until chemotherapy is completed and your white blood count has been restored. However, you can delay reconstruction months or years if you are not fully committed to it or feel uncertain that it is right for you at this time.

Should I have an implant or flap reconstruction?

Consider the pros and cons of each carefully. You have a choice, so don't be talked into something you don't feel comfortable with. Sometimes circumstances aid the decision. For instance, if you are full breasted an implant will not afford symmetry with the other breast. Or, if you smoke and are unable to tolerate flap surgery, you will be limited to an implant.

Will my new breast match my other breast?

If you choose the procedure most appropriate to your circumstances, there is no reason your new breast won't look almost exactly like the other one. But this may take more than one procedure, and it won't happen overnight. It takes time and some follow-up molding and shaping before you have the best possible new breast.

Will my new breast gain or lose weight when I do?

Breasts reconstructed with your own tissue will gain or lose weight with you. A breast implant reconstruction may not — unless your implant is adjustable and can be inflated or deflated with saline at your surgeon's office. Be sure you understand how this works.

What will it look like in ten years?

You certainly want to ask your plastic surgeon what your breast will look like in ten or twenty years. Will it age with you? Will it defy gravity, or will it gradually drop with your other breast? You need to know if you will need adjustments in the future to keep both breasts looking alike. Breasts made with your own tissue generally age like any other part of your body.

May I see pictures and diagrams of the different types of reconstruction?

Any plastic surgeon should show you photographs — before and after — of actual reconstructions. Ask when the photos were taken. You want to see pictures taken right after surgery as well as years later. The surgeon should also give you a simple diagram of where the incisions will be located on your breast and donor sites.

Can you refer me to other patients so I can talk with them about their reconstruction?

The surgeon should be able to give you one or more referrals. If not, ask in your support group and ask your other doctors. Talk with at least one person, and see one — in the flesh. You

want to know what you are getting before you do it. This is
a major undertaking.

How will the procedure affect me physically and emotionally?
This is tough surgery, which can wipe you out and leave you
weak. Loss of blood from major surgery can leave you feeling
run-down and depressed. Recovery is quick, however, and the
more you know about the entire process the better.

Can I donate my own blood to use during and after surgery?
This is standard procedure and a good way to avoid the risk
of infection with hepatitis or AIDS. Your blood is collected a
week or two before surgery and stored in the blood bank. This
gives your body a chance to build up your blood counts so you
are not anemic during surgery.

If I want to change the other breast, what is involved?
Even if you don't think you want to do this, it's a good idea
to know what is involved. You can alter your remaining breast,
making it smaller or larger. The procedure you choose for
reconstruction may be based on the appearance of your remaining breast. You may decide in the future to make changes,
too. Find out about costs and insurance coverage for altera-
tions on the other breast.

When can I go back to work?
After an implant you should be able to resume normal activity
in a week or two. With flap reconstruction, recovery varies,
but you should be able to return to work in four to eight
weeks, and resume more strenuous activity in six months.

Will TRAM reconstruction interfere with future pregnancies?
In the past, the TRAM-flap reconstruction meant there would
not be enough muscle left to support a pregnancy. But more
sophisticated techniques mean this is no longer a problem.

～ 7

Radiation Therapy

Radiation is standard procedure following a lumpectomy, to wipe out any remaining cancer cells from the tumor site. If you have a lumpectomy, you probably have no *detectable* cancer left, but there may be microscopic disease left in the lumpectomy site. Even if the surgeon says, "I got it all," experience shows it is difficult to "get it all" with any real degree of certainty.

In cases of extensive cancer, radiation might also be used with mastectomy. Then it treats the chest wall or the chest wall and skin after mastectomy and reconstruction to reduce the chance of recurrence. Radiation is also used to treat lymph nodes under the arm, beneath the breastbone, or above the collarbone, when the cancer has spread. Depending on the type and extent of your cancer, radiation may be used with chemotherapy or surgery or both.

Generally, if you have a single small cancer no bigger than 1½ inches in diameter (about the size of a peach pit or a Ping-Pong ball), you can probably save your breast with lumpectomy and radiation treatment. Radiation to the breast can be given safely and accurately with an excellent cosmetic result in at least 90 percent of patients treated. In other words, your breast will look and feel very much the way it does now.

Once it has been decided that you may keep your breast,

you must weigh the pluses and minuses of each treatment and consider how important it is for you to keep your breast. You are empowered to make that decision. But feel assured that keeping your breast does not mean your treatment is less effective than mastectomy.

Radiation is meant to mimic mastectomy. Mastectomy removes the whole breast. Therefore, the entire breast is treated with radiation, usually for five weeks, or twenty-five times. At the final phase, treatment is localized to the tumor bed. It is *not* standard therapy to treat only the tumor area.

Radiation treatment after a lumpectomy (and usually a lymph node dissection) for early breast cancer is just as effective as mastectomy in preventing the tumor from coming back where it was. This is accepted scientific fact! Yet some patients and even some doctors still have a hard time understanding this.

There is still a strong belief that the breast must be removed to get all the cancer out. But it has been proven over and over — in radiation and surgical literature, including surveys by the National Institutes of Health — that lumpectomy followed by radiation has the same cure rate as mastectomy. We cannot stress this enough!

How Long Has Radiation Treatment Been in Use?

Radiation therapy has been around for a hundred years — since the discovery of X rays and radium. In fact, breast cancer was one of the first types of cancer to be treated with radiation. But in the early years only low-energy equipment existed, leading to a high complication and low cure rate. During the following years, especially after the 1940s, great strides were made in the development of equipment for treating cancer. Eventually, powerful high-energy radiation machines improved cure rates, and complications decreased.

Since the 1960s, developments in electronics and computers have led to some amazing equipment for diagnosing and treating cancer patients. Normal tissues can now be visualized in relation to cancer in three dimensions. The treatment area can be aligned and positioned for the highest accuracy.

Lumpectomy with radiation has been used to treat breast cancer for the past thirty years. However, it is still more commonly used in the northeastern United States than other areas.

How Radiation Works

Radiation has two functions: to cure cancer and prevent its return, and as a palliative treatment — that is, to kill pain and slow the progress of the disease if it has metastasized to the bone, liver, or brain. It can be used by itself or in combination with surgery, either before or after. Approximately 500 to 1,000 times more energy is used in radiation treatment than with regular X rays. This high dosage from high-energy equipment kills all the cells in its path, good and bad, so they cannot grow and multiply. However, new, healthy cells will replace those lost.

Before Beginning Radiation Treatment

Before your surgery, you will have had a series of tests to see whether the cancer has spread. These may involve a chest X ray, blood tests to check your red and white blood cell and hemoglobin counts, and to determine whether blood liver enzymes are elevated, which could be an early warning of cancer in other parts of the body. A bone scan *may* also have been done.

Your radiologist will review results of all these tests, as well as the tissue slides from your biopsy and your mammogram films. She or he will need to know your medical history and find out if you've had radiation before. Your breast will be physically examined many times in the process. Then you and your doctor can discuss your treatment.

Who Should Not Be Treated with Radiation?

If you have had radiation in the past, or if your cancer or calcifications are widespread in your breast, or if you have a large tumor in a small breast, radiation may not be the best treatment. For example, removing a large tumor from a small breast would involve too much resectioning to restore the contour of the breast. Cosmetic results would generally be poor in these cases.

So, radiation therapy might be inappropriate in these circumstances:

- If you have had radiation to the same breast in the past. Past radiation to the other breast would *not* rule you out.
- If you have had radiation treatment for Hodgkin's disease or have a connective tissue disease like scleroderma, or lupus.
- If you have very large breasts, which may result in less satisfactory cosmetic results with radiation. These patients tend to have some shortening and contracture on the treated side.
- If you have multiple tumors in several areas of your breast.
- If you have extensive calcifications in your breast.

Preliminary Steps: Simulation and Planning

As mentioned, radiation is standard procedure following lumpectomy and/or lymph node dissection. Sometimes it is also given after a mastectomy to make sure all the cancer cells that might have lingered on the chest wall or skin are wiped out.

It is common to wait two weeks after surgery for skin and tissue to heal so there is no opening in the incision before beginning radiation treatment, because radiation can slow the healing process. During that waiting time it is important to exercise your arm so that you have good range of motion before beginning the simulation process. Your surgeon or radiation therapist will show you exercises to do at home.

Your first visits (usually three) to the radiation treatment center will be for *simulation,* a process of measuring and marking — usually with an ordinary felt-tip marker — the precise area to be treated. You may be asked not to wash off the marks for a day or two. The technicians will have you lie on a table with your hand over your head (this is one reason the arm exercises are important) and make sure that you are in the correct position so the oblique beam will treat the breast and not the arm unnecessarily.

You may also be fitted for an alpha cradle, so that each time you lie on the table for treatment, you will be in exactly the same position. This cradle is molded by filling a large plastic bag with a liquid material that solidifies to fit your body contours. Such immobilization devices are not used everywhere. Some hospitals simply use a wedge under your body.

Your physician will probably take Polaroid photos of your breast several times during the process. Such documentation helps follow any changes in the size and appearance of your breast.

A CAT scan may be necessary in the treatment-planning process so that a two- or three-dimensional picture of your breast can be re-created in the computer. This helps the radiologist decide exactly how the radiation will penetrate the breast to avoid exposing too much tissue around your rib and lung.

The next visit is usually for an X ray on the same machine where you will be treated. This documents the treatment area. After the X ray, tattoos will be placed on your breast to mark the pathway for the radiation beam. This does not hurt. The tattoos are permanent, but they are so tiny that you'll hardly notice them. Usually about a dozen tattoos are placed, but this can vary from one institution to another.

However they are done, these markers guide the doctors and technicians in directing the radiation to the proper spot. The radiation will treat you from your collarbone to the fold under your breast and from your breastbone to an area near your underarm.

Minor adjustments may be necessary periodically during

your treatments if your breast has swelled. Don't be alarmed. This is only to ensure accuracy. During the treatment period, your radiation doctor will see and examine you and check your dosages. Breaks in treatment may be necessary if your skin becomes irritated too quickly.

If you have any lymph nodes that have tested positive, your underarm may also be treated.

How Often Do I Receive Radiation and How Long Does It Take?

You will be treated daily from Monday through Friday for five to seven weeks. It takes five weeks to treat the whole breast and then two more weeks for the *boost*, a dose of radiation directed into the tumor bed.

Your daily treatments last less than five minutes and are administered by highly trained and state-licensed technicians. With your upper body bare, you will lie down in your cradle and the technicians will set up the machinery and administer the dose of radiation.

Radiation therapy is strictly regulated by federal and state nuclear regulatory commissions. The total dose of radiation delivered to the breast at most institutions is between 4,500 and 5,000 rads, or cGy, which means centigrays. The daily dose will be between 180 and 200 cGy. A boost dosage of an additional 1,000 to 2,000 cGy is delivered directly to the tumor bed in the last part of the treatment. Dosage varies with the philosophy of the institution. It is believed, however, that a total dose to the tumor bed should be in the range of 6,000 to 6,500 cGy. Increasing the dose beyond this increases complications, and cosmetic results are not as good.

Your doctor will visit you periodically to monitor your treatment. At least once a week your doctor should also examine your breast thoroughly and see how you are feeling. She or he may also photograph your breast to keep a record of your progress.

Does Radiation Treatment Burn?

No. It's painless. You may feel some discomfort lying in the cradle, or in the particular position you must maintain while the radiation is penetrating. Technicians will help you lie down. They will set up the machine to the proper angle. They will look at you once or twice from the computer monitor to be sure you are correctly positioned. Then they will ask you to lie still while they turn on the machine. It is just like getting an X ray. You won't feel a thing. The radiation is sent into your breast for only a few seconds, although you may be in position for five minutes or more. After one to two weeks of treatments your breast may swell and the skin in the treated area may redden, turning any shade from slightly pink to deep red.

What Is the Boost?

The boost is the final phase of radiation treatment, usually given during the last two weeks. A boost delivers a dose of radiation directly to the tumor bed. There are two ways to do this: externally, using the radiation machine, or internally, by implanting radioactive pellets in your breast. Cost and cosmetic results are similar.

External boost. Most women get the external boost, because not every radiation oncologist has the experience to do implants. As was mentioned in the surgery chapter, small metal clips — like staples — are inserted at the margins of the surgical bed (the edges of the area where the tumor was) during the lumpectomy. Don't worry, these clips won't set off metal detectors at the airport! But they will remain in your body forever. These clips define the tumor bed to help the radiation oncologist determine where to deliver the boost. When a CAT scan is done as part of the treatment planning, these metal clips can be seen on the scan and a final radiation field can be very accurately placed, based on their position. The boost dose uses the same type of radiation as your previous treatments. It is just more focused.

The interstitial implant is used more often at university hospitals. It is not a new procedure, nor is it any more or less effective than the external boost. While you are in surgery for your lumpectomy, your radiation oncologist will insert small, hollow plastic tubes in your breast tissue where the tumor was — the area surrounded by the clips. These are conduits for radioactive pellets that are placed the day of surgery and provide the local boost dose. The pellets are left in place for about forty-eight hours and removed before you leave the hospital. Then, two weeks later, overall radiation treatment of the breast starts.

The amount of the radiation dose with the implant is usually the same as with the external boost. Once the boost dose is delivered, the implant can be removed in your room without anesthesia in about ten minutes. However, you are considered radioactive for the forty-eight hours the implants are in your breast. This will not cause sterility or affect any part of your body, but the number of visitors to your room will be limited. Since the isotope is emitting some low-energy X rays, no children under eighteen or pregnant women can come to your room. Other visitors can stay for an hour. Some hospitals place a waist-high lead shield at the side of the bed for the protection of nurses who often deal with radiation and try to limit their exposure. Once the implant is out, there are no restrictions.

The tubes are removed as easily as sutures are removed. This may cause some local discomfort during the removal process. Usually an analgesic such as acetaminophen and codeine is sufficient to alleviate this local discomfort.

Can I Continue to Work While Getting Radiation Treatment?

Most women do, and if you can schedule treatment for mornings or late in the afternoon, you can work with little interruption to your day. It is always best to lead as normal a life as possible during the weeks of treatment. However, radiation can make you tired, so don't expect to function at your full capacity. Rest when you need it.

What Side Effects Can I Expect?

Most women have no problem receiving radiation to the breast. The most common side effects are:

- itchy, dry skin in the treatment area
- reddened skin (mild to deep red)
- breast swelling
- blisters under the breast where the bra rubs

All are temporary and are treated with mild creams and sometimes a break in treatment.

Breast swelling usually resolves itself in up to six months in most women. This is related to the extent of the lymph node dissection and occurs to some extent in most women. This is usually a short-term condition.

How Can I Offset These Side Effects?

Here are some things you can do to feel more comfortable.

- Avoid shaving your underarm on the treatment side.
- Don't use antiperspirant, deodorant, or powder on that side.

- Do not use creams or solutions that contain perfumes, alcohol, or aluminum or other metals.
- Use a mild, aloe-based cream after treatment to soothe dry, itchy skin.
- If blisters form, ask your doctor to recommend treatment for this.
- Wear soft cotton clothing and go braless as often as possible.

Are There Any Long-Term Effects of Radiation?

With careful treatment planning and appropriate doses, fewer than 5 percent of patients experience any long-term side effects, such as rib fracture, a scar on the lung, or inflammation of the lung. Some people are more sensitive than others to radiation, and a future trauma, such as a fall or an auto accident, could cause a rib to fracture more easily than it would normally. There is no way to prevent this, but always X-ray any injury to your chest or ribs.

A few women have developed a sarcoma, a tumor of the soft tissue of the breast, as a result of treatment, but most of these women had been treated on old, low-energy equipment. There is no way of knowing if the malignancy was already developing in their breast, or if it developed because radiation injured the underlying soft tissue of their breast.

When radiation hits the part of the lung directly under the chest wall, it can leave a scar on your lung. This part of the lung needs to be included in the radiation field to make sure all of your breast is treated. This scar shows up in X rays in about 5 percent of patients but is symptomatic in less than this. Someone reading your chest X ray might think you had had pneumonia in the past. Careful treatment planning with CAT is important to minimize the amount of lung area in the radiation field.

Radiation's effect on the heart is extremely rare. It occurs in less than 1 percent of patients, and only if the heart is directly within the radiation field. It could cause some scarring or possibly increase the risk of atherosclerosis.

The risk of getting cancer again as a result of radiation is negligible. There is no evidence that radiation on one breast will increase the risk of breast cancer on the opposite side. Nor is there any evidence that it increases the risk of any other cancer, such as lymphoma.

If you are receiving chemotherapy with certain cytotoxic drugs, such as Adriamycin or methotrexate, at the same time as radiation, your skin may react to radiation more intensely and this could result in a less than perfect cosmetic effect. But these drugs can be omitted while you are receiving radiation treatment.

If lymph node areas are treated with radiation, there is a possibility of damage to the nerves underlying the arm, but this is also rare. Tingling sensation and weakness can occur in the arm and hand. Another risk of treating the underarm lymph node area is the increased likelihood of arm swelling, or lymphedema. There is a 20 percent risk of swelling as a result of radiation, and it may become a long-term condition. However, it can be treated and kept in check so that it does not disrupt your life — or your appearance. (See Chapter 14.)

What Will My Breast Look Like After Radiation?

With state-of-the-art radiation equipment, 90 percent of patients believe their breast looks and feels similar to the untreated breast, though the treated breast usually seems slightly firmer. As one fifty-year-old woman quipped, "Now I have a twenty-year-old breast and a fifty-year-old breast!" The majority of patients report excellent cosmetic results.

It may take as long as a year for the breast to return to its normal state. It may remain slightly red for a few months, and larger than normal. As mentioned earlier, cosmetic results depend largely on how much breast tissue is removed. If a large tumor is removed from a small breast, the cosmetic results can be less satisfactory, because a greater proportion of the breast will have been removed.

With any size breast the cosmetic results can be less than satisfactory if too much of the tissue has been removed. That is why it is so important to find a surgeon with experience in treating breast cancer. Determining just how much tissue to remove without compromising either your recurrence rate or the cosmetic result requires precision and sensitivity.

What Follow-up Care Will I Need?

When radiation therapy is completed, expect to have a routine checkup within two months. This will include physical examination of the breast to check the aftereffects of treatment. Then visit your radiation oncologist at regular six-month intervals for five years.

You should also see your surgeon at six-month intervals, but be sure to stagger your appointments so you receive a breast examination every three or four months. You may also alternate with your medical oncologist if you are taking hormone or cytotoxic chemotherapy. This close follow-up procedure continues for five years, while the potential for recurrence is highest. After that you visit everyone — radiologist, oncologist, surgeon — annually.

Six months after completing radiation therapy you should have a bilateral (both breasts) mammogram. The mammogram of the treated breast will continue at six-month intervals for two years and then once a year. The mammogram of the untreated breast can continue at regular yearly intervals.

Ask your radiation oncologist, your surgeon, or your medical oncologist if you will need a bone scan at yearly intervals, along with tumor marker studies, including a CA15-3 and CEA. These are blood tests that detect certain antigens made by tumor cells. Routine pelvic and rectal examinations by your gynecologist are also important. You may want to see a physical therapist if you need more mobility in your arm. And, always, always do your monthly breast self-exams.

Obviously, the extent and frequency of follow-up testing depend upon the extent and degree of your breast cancer. All of this testing may turn out to be negative for the rest of your life. And in the majority of early breast cancer cases it does. But the point is, never leave it to chance. If you monitor your health, you will find any recurrence early enough to treat it and save your life.

How Do I Find the Best Place to Have Radiation Therapy?

Radiation therapy is most often done in big city hospitals, teaching hospitals, and comprehensive cancer centers (hospitals that treat only cancer); and it is more commonly done in the Northeast, although excellent centers can be found in all parts of the United States. There are many ways to find a radiation oncologist and radiation center. Your physician can refer you, or you can call the American Cancer Society, the National Cancer Institute, or the American College of Radiology. Support groups, libraries, and hotlines are also good sources of information. (See Appendix 4.)

Big city teaching hospitals and comprehensive cancer centers often provide better treatment because they treat so many more patients, attract more experienced physicians, and use up-to-date equipment. Ask if a simulator is available for treatment planning, along with a high-energy 4–6 megavolt photon beam with electron capability. You'll want to know that there is a CAT scanner available and a physicist on staff to handle problems that may arise with the equipment. If your surgeon does not feel the need to send you to a radiation oncologist experienced in breast cancer, it may be wise to go find one yourself. You may feel better with a second opinion. Call the breast cancer information groups listed in Appendix 4.

Look around. The treatment *is not* an emergency. So move with deliberate speed, and don't make any snap judgments based on emotions. Learn as much as you can first, so you will feel more comfortable and be ready to make an educated decision. Take a friend or loved one with you on interviews and consultations. Take notes. Bring a tape recorder!

What Does Radiation Therapy Cost?

A complete program of radiation therapy for breast cancer can cost as much as $30,000 in a large medical center in the Northeast. This includes treatment planning and thirty-five treatments. Most of that is a technical fee, and about a third is the professional fee. Most medical insurance covers this cost. Medicare covers 80 percent of the cost and Medicaid covers it all.

✔ **Questions to Ask Before Deciding on Radiation Therapy**

These questions are meant to help you interview physicians and other healthcare professionals so that you can feel secure about your treatment decisions. Some of these questions have no clear-cut answers, some do. But ask anyway! For instance, you don't need to understand how the machinery works, but there are manufacturing standards. Most hospitals conform to these standards, but sometimes there are exceptions. Take this book with you and ask the questions you want to know about. It is your responsibility to get the best treatment you can. So don't be bashful!

Do you have high-energy machinery (4–6 megavolts) with electron capability?

If the machinery is new, it probably meets these standards; however, it is still wise to ask.

Do you have CAT simulation and planning and a physicist on staff?

If the answer is no, it means they cannot get the optimum precision required for applying radiation to your breast.

Is the radiation delivered by licensed technicians?

Radiation technicians must be licensed by the state.

What is the dosage of radiation used for breast cancer?

It should be somewhere between 4,500 and 5,000 rads.

What type of boost will you use?

Electron (external) boost and implant (internal) boost are equally effective, but not all hospitals are equipped to handle the internal boost.

How often will I see my radiation oncologist during the course of treatment?

At least once a week during the course of treatment for a thorough visit. But a resident or attending physician should be available to you anytime you need one or have a question.

How long will I have to wait for treatment every day?

Scheduling should be done so that you wait no longer than half an hour, and more commonly, only a few minutes.

May I see some photos of other women who have been treated here?

There should be no objection, because faces are not usually photographed and no privacy is invaded. Look at the cosmetic results; note any deformity, skin changes, asymmetry with the other breast, and placement of incisions.

What kind of follow-up care can I expect?

Be sure the treatment center provides thorough follow-up care. Ask if they include blood tests like the CA15-3 and CEA. These test for antigens in your blood that may indicate remaining cancer cells.

Will my insurance take care of simulation and planning, treatment, follow-up care, and any related expenses?

It's very important that you understand the cost of everything, so that you don't get billed later for things like the cost of making the cradle, or find out that your insurance does not cover follow-up exams. Always check with your insurance company, too.

~ 8

Chemotherapy: Improved Drugs, Fewer Side Effects

Chemotherapy works. It kills cancer cells. It also kills normal cells, and that's why the side effects are so potent. But the normal cells grow back, and there are ways to cope with side effects. Chemotherapy is the use of any chemical agent, such as drugs, steroids, or hormones, inside the body for a system-wide treatment. You may take these drugs in the form of pills, or you may receive them via injections or intravenous infusions. Chemotherapy is used to cure cancer or keep it from spreading. For breast cancer it commonly includes two kinds of chemical agents:

- cytotoxic drugs used before or after surgery to kill cancer cells and shrink tumors, or
- chemohormonal agents, like tamoxifen, to prevent the cancer from coming back

Chemotherapy Before or After Surgery

Until the mid-1980s, chemotherapy was used only if a woman had positive lymph nodes, and then only after surgery. Then we started using chemotherapy as a way to shrink larger tumors *before* surgery, with dramatic results. Now there are two ways to use chemotherapy: neoadjuvant, which means before other treatment, and adjuvant therapy, which is combined with or follows local treatment, such as surgery or radiation. In these situations, there is no evidence of tumor elsewhere in the system and the drugs are used as protection. Chemotherapy is also used to eradicate or control the cancer if it recurs elsewhere in the body.

Because no two people react in just the same way to any particular drug, each patient is evaluated individually. The treatments are usually given in the doctor's office, although in some cases an overnight hospital stay may be prescribed. The frequency of treatment is up to your chemotherapist, but it is usually given in cycles — such as once every three or four weeks — so that your body has a drug-free period to repair the normal cells.

Chemotherapy has long been associated with nausea, hair loss, and other difficult side effects, but these are not the same for everyone. Some women experience only mild reactions. Generally, the most powerful side effects of nausea and vomiting last for a few days after each treatment, then subside. Hair loss (alopecia) and fatigue may last until the end of the treatments. The good news is, chemotherapy is no longer prescribed for two years. Now, it's given for three to six months, and there are effective drugs to combat some of the side effects.

Who Gets Cytotoxic Chemotherapy, and When?

Every case of breast cancer is unique because there are so many variables. Generally, if you are at high risk for systemic disease, with a tumor over 1–2 centimeters (⅓–¾ inch) in diameter, with one or more positive lymph nodes or an aggressive (high-grade) cancer, you may be treated with chemotherapy. When planning chemotherapy treatment, your medical oncologist will consider many factors, including your age, whether you are pre- or postmenopausal (or pregnant), the size and type of your tumor and its grade (aggressiveness), and the number of lymph nodes involved. Other indicators can include the results of many of the pathology studies of cell behavior.

Weighing benefits and risks. Always be aware of the health benefits and risks of adjuvant chemotherapy. These risks are constantly being studied by the medical profession. Our goal for the future is the development of a risk profile system — a list of prognostic indicators — to estimate prognosis on an individual basis. Four major international trials are now in progress to look at adjuvant chemotherapy in node-negative women. These studies are evaluating tamoxifen as well as cytotoxic chemotherapy. Ask your oncologist about these studies so you can keep current.

Chemotherapy and fertility. Because chemotherapy could force you into menopause, you need to consider carefully whether or not you want to be pregnant in the future. If your lymph nodes are positive and you are premenopausal, you need chemotherapy for sure. Often, you will spontaneously resume menses several months after completing chemotherapy, but not always. There is considerable controversy among physicians about giving chemotherapy to young women with negative lymph nodes. Studies of treated versus untreated groups show the same survival, but women who had chemotherapy showed a 15 percent improvement in *disease-free* survival. This means systemic recurrence is delayed by one or two years. This is something only you can decide once you have all the facts. The only difference in menopause brought on by chemotherapy is that it is an abrupt change rather than a gradual one. You must suddenly deal with an aspect of your development you hadn't expected to confront yet.

Chemotherapy with surgery. If you have Stage III cancer — locally advanced or inflammatory breast cancer that has not metastasized to other organs — you may need an initial treatment with chemotherapy for about three months before surgery.

This is called neoadjuvant (or induction) chemotherapy. Some doctors prescribe it for six or nine months, but this depends on how much the tumor shrinks or responds. Neoadjuvant chemotherapy aims to shrink a tumor by at least 50 percent before surgery is performed. Tumor reduction is also used as a barometer. If the breast tumor does *not* shrink, then any unseen tumors that may be in the body have not shrunk either. It is believed that the response of the tumor in the breast indicates the overall response of the body to the drugs. Once the tumor is smaller, surgery can proceed. Then chemotherapy resumes after surgery for an average of six months.

Chemotherapy and radiation. Chemotherapy commonly follows lumpectomy and radiation in the treatment of early breast cancer. The type of chemotherapy is determined by the prognostic factors and tumor characteristics. Tamoxifen is commonly used in older women with early disease and does not have the side effects of cytotoxic drugs. Patients with more than four positive nodes or a tumor site without clean margins may also need cytotoxic chemotherapy after surgery and radiation.

For women with early breast cancer with clean nodes — Stages I and II — chemotherapy can be given during or after radiation therapy. We have to watch drugs like Adriamycin and methotrexate, which can make the skin reaction from radiation more intense. Your doctor may eliminate the drug until after radiation treatment ends. If they are given separately, your treatment team must decide which comes first. Which risk is greater — local or systemic?

For locally advanced, Stage III, breast cancer, any of these combinations of treatment may apply:

- chemotherapy, then mastectomy plus or minus radiation, then chemotherapy
- chemotherapy, then lumpectomy and axillary dissection plus radiation, then chemotherapy
- chemotherapy, then radiation, then chemotherapy

Obviously, for Stage III disease, it is important that you be seen by all doctors for a multidisciplinary approach to treatment. Recent evidence indicates that carefully selected patients with large breast masses or positive nodes in the axilla may respond to neoadjuvant chemotherapy and then have the option of breast conservation with radiation, instead of mastectomy. After about two years of observation, results for this particular group as of early 1994 seem comparable to the results attained by treatment with mastectomy.

Which Cytotoxic Drugs Are Used for Breast Cancer?

Cytotoxic drugs have a variety of mechanisms of action. For instance, Cytoxan (cyclophosphamide), an alkylating agent, prevents cancer cells from multiplying. The antimetabolites methotrexate and 5-fluorouracil (5-FU) trick the cells into absorbing them by blocking nutrients from your food. This action essentially starves the cells. All cells. The antitumor antibiotics like Adriamycin (doxorubicin) interfere with the cells' DNA to inhibit growth. So these drugs either shrink tumors or slow down or stop cell growth. They can be used alone or in combination, and for a variety of time periods. Combinations try to take advantage of the different mechanisms and thereby kill the most cells. Which drugs are used and how they are administered depends on your type of cancer, prognosis, your doctor, and your own preference.

The drugs discussed below are the ones most often used for breast cancer chemotherapy, and are most commonly used in combination. That is, one at a time in a calculated sequence. A second line of drugs includes mitomycin (Mutamycin), which is similar to Adriamycin, along with vincristine (Oncovin), vinblastine (Velban), thiotepa, and the new drugs taxol and RU-486. Taxol has been approved by the Food and Drug Administration for use in treating breast cancer, but as of this writing RU-486 has not.

Methotrexate has been in use since 1947 and is administered by pill or injection. The chance of developing kidney and bladder problems, most typically cystitis, is high with this drug. This can be avoided by drinking lots of fluids. Methotrexate affects your skin, too, causing rashes and photosensitivity, so it's best to stay out of the sun. Mouth and lip sores are also common. Because this drug affects your blood platelets and the ability of your blood to coagulate, don't take aspirin or aspirin products, which thin your blood. Methotrexate can also cause nausea and vomiting, and in severe cases, can lead to anorexia.

Fluorouracil (5-FU) is given by injection and has been associated with the entire gamut of side effects: nausea and vomiting, anorexia, hair loss, rash, itching, diarrhea, fever and chills, bruising and bleeding.

Cyclophosphamide (Cytoxan) has been in use since 1960. You may notice darkening of your fingernails with this one, as well as anorexia, hair loss, nausea and vomiting, fever and chills, mouth sores, jaundice, and frequent urination. Drink plenty of fluids.

Doxorubicin (Adriamycin), in use since 1974, is sometimes used with more aggressive tumors, with four or more positive lymph nodes, or in younger premenopausal women. It can cause urine to turn red, but this is not blood. This drug can affect your heart — it is cardiotoxic — so if you notice an irregular heartbeat, or if your feet swell, call your doctor. Hair loss generally occurs. Pain at the injection site — a common complaint — can mean that some of the drug has leaked out of the vein. It is very irritating to the surrounding soft tissue and can cause a slough of the skin if leaks occur.

The New Drugs: Taxol and RU-486

Taxol is a new and effective drug used to treat ovarian and breast cancer. It comes from the bark of the rare and endangered Pacific yew tree. Its cost is high since it takes as many as six 100-year-old trees to treat one patient. However, re-searchers have produced a synthetic drug, taxotere, with the same structure and function that is as effective, and easier to tolerate. Taxol prevents cells from dividing, and so far has been approved for use in treating ovarian cancer. A nation-wide clinical trial, sponsored by the National Cancer Institute in 1993, is under way with four thousand women with breast, ovarian, and other cancers. If the results are as positive as we hope, taxol should become more widely used for breast cancer.

The other new drug, RU-486, the so-called French abortion pill, inhibits the growth of breast cancer cells. The drug, approved in December 1993 for use in treating breast cancer, works much like tamoxifen in blocking the interaction of cancer cells with hormones, but it is more directed against progesterone. Canadian researchers began large-scale clinical trials with breast cancer patients, and we should know more about it before the end of the century.

For the latest information on drugs call:

- **American Cancer Society**   800-ACS-2345
  Your local chapter should have the latest information on drugs.
- **NABCO Hotline**   212-719-0154
  Ask for their fact sheets on particular drugs or treatments.
- **NCI Cancer Information Hotline**   800-4-CANCER
  They have the latest information on new drugs.

How Is Chemotherapy Administered?

Chemotherapy can be as simple as taking a couple of pills every day, or visiting your doctor's office for an injection. Or, you may be hospitalized overnight for an intravenous infusion, which slowly releases the drugs into your bloodstream for better tolerance.

Most commonly, treatment is administered every three to four weeks in your oncologist's office. A specially trained nurse or physician's assistant injects the medication directly into your vein (intravenous). Often a small metal "port" with a soft plastic tube connecting to your vein is implanted under your skin near your collarbone. The chemotherapist can attach a catheter to the port and feed the drugs directly into your bloodstream from an IV bag. In the past, ports were used only after veins in the arm and hand were exhausted. Now they are often placed at the beginning of treatment, to avoid exhausting the arm and hand veins — and to make it easier to take the drugs.

Implanting the port is an outpatient procedure using local anesthesia with intravenous sedation. The vein under the collarbone is accessed with a needle, then a dilator is used to place the catheter in the vein. The procedure is monitored under fluoroscopy to ensure correct placement in the superior vena cava — the main vein that brings blood to your heart. A metal port is secured to your muscle and your skin is sutured closed. Having a port allows you, in some cases, to have a therapist come to your home to administer chemotherapy. Sometimes the ports can also be used to draw blood samples.

For the first day or two after you receive your dose of chemotherapy, you will feel the side effects most strongly, especially nausea and loss of appetite, and then these will taper off. That's why the doses are cyclical. This gives you a chance to recuperate and repair your cells before the next dose. About three weeks after you start the cycle, your blood counts may drop. This is monitored by your chemotherapist. If your counts become too low — particularly your white blood cells, which guard against infection — your chemotherapist will be able to warn you.

How Do I Know If Chemotherapy Is Working?

Some women think that if they have no side effects the cytotoxic drugs are not doing their job. Not true. The degree of your side effects is no indication of whether or not the chemotherapy is working. Physicians in this field strive to administer chemotherapy with a minimum of adverse effects. Your chemotherapist monitors your progress with periodic blood tests, physical examinations, X rays, or computer scans. These screenings also monitor possible toxicity to other organs. Physical exams and lab tests may be done each time you go in for your treatment. Ask your doctor what the tests are showing, including the blood tumor markers. Most physicians have equipment that can process many tests quickly with one vial of your blood. The usual laboratory tests include the CBC (complete blood count: white cells, red cells, and platelets), SMA12 (which is a set of twelve tests that look at liver and kidney function), and tumor markers (CEA, CA15-3, CA125). Monitoring white blood cell and platelet count during treatment is vital. A low white count could mean you are increasingly at risk for infection, and a low platelet count would mean your blood won't clot. Normal white blood cell count range is between 4,000 and 11,000; platelet count is between 140,000 and 400,000.

Coping with Side Effects

The worst side effects are the gastrointestinal problems created by the cytotoxic drugs. You can't eat because you are nauseous and the smell of food makes it worse. Even food you once loved turns your stomach. Sores in your mouth hurt when you swallow. For most women, the nausea feels like mild morning sickness, and nibbling on crackers may ease the effect. The intensity of your reaction to chemotherapy is impossible to predict. But, assuming you will feel sick part of the time, or have some mouth sores, there are ways to get through it.

Nausea. First, ask your oncologist for medications to help the nausea. Zofran, for instance, is very good at this and can be given intravenously. Compazine and Reglan are given orally. Some medications are available as rectal suppositories if you are too nauseous to keep oral drugs down. Take these *before* the symptoms strike. If your symptoms are really severe, your doctor may recommend a sedative so you can relax or sleep through the most difficult period.

Hypnosis or biofeedback may also be useful. Some women have learned relaxation techniques and visualization; they visualize the cytotoxic drugs killing their cancer cells. A derivative of marijuana in pill form can be legally prescribed by some physicians, and it is frequently used to combat nausea during chemotherapy.

Keep in mind that the side effects are strongest right after you get your treatment. In a couple of days, you will feel better and gradually improve until you get the next dose. And the cycle begins again. Meanwhile, you must eat to keep up your strength, and to keep your normal cells regenerating. Here are some ideas to help you keep eating while your gastrointestinal tract is rebelling.

- Eat high-calorie, low-volume foods such as ice cream. High-fat foods have more than twice as many calories per gram as protein and carbohydrates. Don't worry about your fat intake now. After chemotherapy treatment you can work on a low-fat, high-fiber diet. Right now you want to concentrate on *not* losing weight.

- Drink at least eight glasses of fluid — water and juices — every day to keep your body well hydrated. This is tough if you are nauseated. Try clear broth to get the fluid and some nutrition at the same time.

- Limit alcohol intake.

- Eat high-protein foods like meat, fish, and dairy products, to help repair your damaged normal cells.

- Eat smaller, more frequent meals.

- Try high-calorie drinks like milk shakes or supplements like Ensure.

- Snack every hour. You need calories. Carry snacks such as dried fruit or plain crackers with you.

- There is a helpful booklet called *Eating Hints: Recipes and Tips for Better Nutrition During Cancer Treatment,* which you can get from the National Cancer Institute. (See Appendix 4.)

    If you are *really* nauseous:

- Try sips of water first, then a little more.
- Eat only one bite of something until you are gradually able to eat more.
- Chew your food well.
- Eat food at room temperature so the aromas don't affect you.
- Avoid big meals.
- Avoid carbonated beverages.
- Suck on hard candies if you can. Jelly beans and dried candied ginger also help.
- Avoid heavy sweets and fried or fatty foods.
- Breathe deeply and slowly when you feel nauseated.
- Wear loose clothing.
- Don't lie down right after you eat. Keep your head elevated.

If you have mouth sores keep your mouth as clean as possible to prevent infection. Brush your teeth gently with a very soft brush after each meal. If the brush bothers you, use a cotton swab.

Here's a mouthwash you can make to ease the sores and help keep your mouth clean.

> 1 teaspoon of salt
> 1 teaspoon of baking soda
> 1 quart of warm water

Mix together, and rinse your mouth several times during the day to remove bacteria and soothe the delicate tissue inside your mouth.

If sores are painful enough to prevent you from swallowing and eating, ask your doctor about nonprescription lozenges and sprays such as Cepacol, to numb your mouth and throat so that you will be able to eat. Your doctor can also prescribe Xylocaine, a local anesthetic, and Benadryl elixir, which you can add to the mixture above. Boil the water and add salt first, and when that mixture is cool, add the baking soda plus three tablespoons of viscous Xylocaine and two tablespoons of Benadryl elixir. Swish this around in your mouth. This should provide some relief. Otherwise:

- Eat soft and soothing foods like applesauce, ice cream, or frozen yogurt.
- Avoid high-acid foods like citrus fruits and tomato sauce.
- Avoid very hot or very cold foods and liquids.
- Avoid salt; it hurts.
- Drink through a straw.
- Suck on ice chips, popsicles, or sugarless candy, or chew sugarless gum.
- See your dentist for gum care and ask for special toothpaste if your teeth and gums are sore.
- Don't smoke!

If you have diarrhea for more than twenty-four hours, or if you are getting painful cramps, let your doctor know. There may be medications to help ease this condition. Otherwise, you can try these:

- Drink plenty of room-temperature fluids like water, apple juice, weak tea, or ginger ale that has gone flat.
- Try the BRAT diet: banana, rice, applesauce, toast.
- Eat low-fiber foods like white bread, rice or noodles, ripe bananas, cottage cheese, yogurt, eggs, potatoes, pureed vegetables, poultry without the skin, fish.
- Avoid high-fiber foods like raw vegetables, beans, nuts, whole-grain breads and cereals.
- Avoid fried, greasy, or highly spiced foods.

- Avoid milk products if these seem to make it worse.
- Avoid tea, coffee, alcohol, and sweets.

If you are constipated from the chemotherapy, from other medications like narcotics, or from the lack of exercise when you are not feeling well, ask your doctor if you should take any medications for this. Otherwise, these may help:

- Drink warm and hot fluids such as coffee, tea, or soup to get things moving.
- Eat lots of high-fiber foods like whole-grain breads and cereals, raw vegetables, fresh and dried fruits.
- Take a natural stool softener such as Metamucil daily to help maintain regularity.
- Try to get some exercise. Walking is good.

Infection is more likely during chemotherapy, because your white blood cells are being devastated. These cells fight infection, and if they are depleted or too low at the time when the next cycle of chemotherapy is to start, then chemotherapy may be postponed until your white cells regenerate. Here are some ways to avoid infection:

- Take good care of your teeth. Teeth and gums are very susceptible to infections because of the amount of bacteria in the mouth.
- Stay away from people who are sick with colds or flu or other communicable diseases.
- Avoid crowds.
- Wash your hands often.
- Clean cuts and bruises immediately with antiseptic, warm water, and soap.
- If you suspect infection, call your doctor. You may need antibiotics.

Skin and nails. Some drugs make skin more sensitive to irritation or to sunburn, and it may be advisable to avoid direct sun. Ask your doctor to recommend creams or lotions to use if you develop severe dry skin, blotchy skin, a rash, or an acnelike condition that is quite common. Your skin may become pale or even discolored. Use a soft, creamy cleanser instead of soap for a while, and experiment with makeup. The American Cancer Society's Look Good, Feel Better program can give you information on skin care and makeup. (Check Appendix 4 for the phone number.) Your nails may also become brittle and break easily, so keep them short.

Fatigue or anemia. You will be tired from chemotherapy simply because your body is under attack by medication. Don't fight it. Rest when you feel tired, and don't try to tackle a normal schedule if you are not up to it. If you also feel weak or dizzy and have chills and shortness of breath, you may be anemic. Your bone marrow's ability to make the red blood cells that carry oxygen around your body may be hampered by chemotherapy, or by blood loss during surgery, and anemia can occur. Your doctor needs to know about this. In the meantime:

- Get plenty of rest.
- Ask for help from family and friends when you need it.
- Get up slowly from a reclining position to prevent dizziness.
- Try to eat well and include iron-rich foods like green leafy vegetables, raisins, and red meats, especially liver, in your diet.
- Take a multivitamin with iron. Chewable children's vitamins are easier to tolerate if you are nauseous. Ask your pharmacist about this.

Hair loss is called alopecia. If your doctor tells you that a loss is certain, then go get a wig before your hair falls out. Chemotherapy can give you the ultimate bad hair day! Some women prefer to shave their heads rather than watch their hair fall out gradually. If you only have thinning hair, it will be less obvious with a short haircut. With a wig or turban, you can create a new look for yourself. A few women have made a powerful and unique statement by going around bald! If you are more conventional, there are methods of caring for your hair as it thins.

- Don't shampoo too often.
- Use very mild or baby shampoos.
- Use wide-tooth combs.
- Try not to blow-dry.
- Get frequent haircuts to keep the shape.
- Don't use any color or perm your hair until it comes back completely.

Because chemotherapy affects your hair follicles, your hair may break off near your scalp, leaving your scalp tender. You may also lose body hair, including your eyebrows and lashes. Just keep in mind that your hair will grow back — everywhere — when the treatment is over. You could be surprised with a slightly different color and texture in your regrowth. Straight hair has come back wavy or curly in the majority of cases, and gray hair may return a darker color.

Wigs are widely available in specialty and department stores, as well as special stores that cater to cancer patients. A human-hair wig looks great, but it is expensive and you must wash and style it. It can be permed, however, and is very natural looking. It can cost from $800 to $1500. Artificial-hair wigs are cheaper and easier to care for. Call several places for prices. Some cater to chemotherapy patients and have private facilities for consultation.

The cost of a wig for use during chemotherapy is usually covered by medical insurance. There may be limits as to how many you can buy, however. A wig is also a tax-deductible medical expense. For more sources of wigs, try these:

- Y-ME has a wig bank for women who cannot afford to buy them.
- Your local American Cancer Society (ACS) chapter should have a list of wig suppliers. Some chapters have wig banks for women with limited incomes.
- Look Good, Feel Better has a program of workshops available in many communities to show you how to use makeup, scarves, and wigs during chemotherapy. They work in cooperation with the ACS.
- The NABCO resource catalog lists many sources for wigs.

If Side Effects Become Severe

When you feel lousy, it's not always easy to figure out when lousy becomes intolerable. Always ask your doctor if you suspect that a side effect is too intense, or you develop an unexpected side effect. Talk with women in your support group. This is another good reason for that network. You can compare notes about treatment and side effects. Call your oncologist if any of the following occur:

- fever, chills, or cold or flu symptoms
- redness or swelling around the injection site
- profuse bleeding from a cut or abrasion
- bruising easily
- blood in urine or stool, black stool, or profuse diarrhea
- nausea and vomiting
- becoming anorexic
- change in mental status
- unsteadiness, dizziness, fainting

Can I Continue to Work During Chemotherapy Treatment?

This is really up to you and will depend on how much and what kind of chemotherapy you are getting. If you feel up to it, then by all means go to work, especially if you like your job! But you will be tired. Try to schedule your chemotherapy treatments late in the day or just before the weekend so that you can rest before returning to work. Adjust your work schedule if you can. Some employers may be required by federal and state law to allow you to work a flexible or part-time schedule. You may also be able to arrange to work at home. Your local American Cancer Society chapter has booklets about federal and state law — including a copy of the recent Americans with Disabilities law. For information about your area, consult:

- your hospital social worker
- your congressional and state representatives
- the National Cancer Institute guide *Facing Forward,* which has work-related information

Planning Around Your Good Days

You may want to track your chemotherapy on a big calendar and plan your life around your treatment cycles. This way you will know when you can eat what you like, or when you will be too nauseous to attend a dinner party. If you have an important business meeting or family wedding and want to be at your best and enjoy yourself, you may be able to plan your treatments around your schedule. Chemotherapy can be flexible. Talk with your doctor. Together you can work out a schedule. You can even arrange for chemotherapy at other facilities if you are going on an extended trip.

Do Sex and Chemotherapy Mix?

Your sex drive may not be up to par, but only temporarily. This is like everything else in your life now. If you feel up to it, then do it. Affection is very important to you right now. If you and your partner can talk openly and honestly about your feelings, it will certainly help you cope with treatment. It's important to communicate with your partner — and with your doctor if you are worried about possible injury. Be cautious about birth control, because chemotherapy will affect your menstrual cycle.

What Is Tamoxifen and How Does It Work?

Tamoxifen is a hormone blocker. Most women have no side effects at all from its use, except for some weight gain, hot flashes, and other menopausal symptoms. Tamoxifen is also known by the brand name Nolvadex and has been used since 1974 to treat women with advanced breast cancer. Now it is used as adjuvant chemotherapy for early-stage breast cancer, to reduce the chance of recurrence, particularly in postmenopausal women with positive estrogen receptors. In the future it may be used as preventive therapy for women at risk.

Tamoxifen is sometimes called an antiestrogen, because it blocks the estrogen receptor and thereby the ability of any cancer cells to use estrogen to grow. Tamoxifen is believed to reduce by at least 20 percent the risk of recurrence in the same breast within ten years and reduce by 50 percent the risk of a new cancer in the opposite breast. We will have a more accurate accounting when the results of a national clinical trial now under way are in.

Tamoxifen is most commonly used following lumpectomy and radiation treatment in postmenopausal women with hormone-positive (ER/PR) tumors. If you have more than four positive lymph nodes, you may get cytotoxic chemotherapy *and* tamoxifen. If you are premenopausal with hormone-positive tumors, tamoxifen may also be used for long-term maintenance. If your estrogen receptors are negative, tamoxifen is unlikely to work. (Studies show it works only 5 percent of the time in these cases.)

Standard treatment is two 10-milligram pills a day — morning and night — for five years or for life. When the five-year tamoxifen trial conducted by the National Cancer Institute is finished in 1998 we will know more. The trial aims to test the effectiveness of tamoxifen in reducing the incidence of breast cancer in the opposite breast in women who have breast cancer on one side, and in acting as a preventive in healthy women at risk because of a family history of breast cancer. If a woman has had minimal side effects from taking tamoxifen for five years, she might continue taking it for life.

Tamoxifen doesn't force you into menopause, although you may have some of the same symptoms that occur during menopause. Irregular periods, vaginal discharge or bleeding, and irritation of the skin around the vagina have been frequently reported. As with menopause, not all women get these symptoms. Discuss these symptoms with your oncologist and gynecologist. If you are premenopausal, your ovaries will continue to act normally and produce estrogen — sometimes more than usual. Other women will experience hot flashes and menopausal symptoms. Tamoxifen can increase fertility, so be careful about birth control. But don't use birth control pills, because that would change the effects of the drug. If you are postmenopausal, tamoxifen can act almost like estrogen-replacement therapy by reducing your risk of heart disease and osteoporosis. This seems paradoxical, and we are still unable to explain exactly why it works that way. Unfortunately, you will probably have hot flashes, sweats, mood swings, depression, and weight gain. But as with everything else, we are all unique; some women report no symptoms whatever.

The Short- and Long-Term Side Effects of Tamoxifen

The side effects of tamoxifen are much less severe than those of cytotoxic chemotherapy. Hot flashes and weight gain are the most common, with bone pain, skin rashes, or vaginal discharge or bleeding affecting a few women. Tamoxifen is a very powerful appetite stimulant, and women report gaining as much as thirty-five pounds, although ten to fifteen pounds is average. You'll have to work at keeping the weight off with a good diet and exercise regimen.

Eye changes. Call your doctor if your vision is blurred. There have been rare reports of retinal changes — thought to be reversible — and it is important to let your ophthalmologist know you are taking tamoxifen. Have your eyes checked annually.

Endometrial cancer. Over the long term, you have a five times greater risk of getting endometrial cancer, the same as the risk to women taking estrogen-replacement therapy. Biopsy of your uterus lining (endometrium) can detect early signs of endometrial cancer. This cancer, by the way, is less aggressive than ovarian cancer and if detected early can be cured with hysterectomy. Annual pap smears and gynecological exams are mandatory for anyone who has had cancer. If you notice any spotting or vaginal discharge, call your gynecologist for evaluation.

Blood clots. The risk of blood clots — thrombophlebitis — from tamoxifen is the same as the risk from birth control pills or estrogen-replacement therapy. Blood clots are rarely fatal if caught quickly and treated, usually with blood-thinning medications. Treatment with blood thinners may require short hospitalization to stabilize you. If you notice pain or swelling in your legs, call your oncologist. If you are also receiving cytotoxic chemotherapy along with tamoxifen, you may be at increased risk for blood clots, but this is extremely rare.

Another drug used as hormone therapy, megestrol (Megace), is sometimes given to patients who have too many side effects from tamoxifen, or who have metastatic disease.

Who Should Give Me Chemotherapy?

A medical oncologist is a doctor of internal medicine who specializes in the treatment of cancer using medications as therapy. Because an internist is trained to understand internal systems, like the cardiovascular, pulmonary, endocrine, digestive, and renal systems, he or she is best able to know how chemotherapy affects those systems. Again, always interview your potential doctors first. Treatment philosophies can differ in the uses of chemotherapy for breast cancer, too, so choose a therapist with whom you feel confident and who has experience with breast cancer. Your medical oncologist will talk with you and other members of your treatment team, and examine you thoroughly before administering your chemotherapy. Your oncologist will study your medical reports, especially the pathology report, to find out how your particular cancer cells can be expected to react to drugs. Some cancer cells are drug resistant.

Find out what your options are. There may be more than one way to go with the chemotherapy. For instance, will your doctor want to use one drug or a combination of drugs? How will the therapy be done? In the office or the hospital? How often? What are the side effects?

Your oncologist will monitor your progress with periodic checkups during therapy and then for a period of time after treatment ends. Visits during treatment may include checking your weight and blood pressure, doing a physical examination, and testing your blood to see if the chemotherapy is working and to monitor for possible toxicity. Unless you have advanced disease in which you can use an X ray or CAT scan to see the tumor shrink, there really is nothing to monitor other than your blood counts or your side effects from chemotherapy.

To find out more about medical oncologists experienced with breast cancer, the following resources are available.

- **The Chemotherapy Foundation**   212-213-9292
Ask for a list of certified oncologists in your area and their booklet on chemotherapy and breast cancer.
- **NABCO Hotline**   212-719-0154
Fact sheets about chemotherapy in English and Spanish.
- **NCI Cancer Information Service
Hotline**   800-4-CANCER
Ask for the Community Clinical Oncology Program list of seventy-five medical centers in thirty-four states selected by NCI to participate in the newest chemotherapy protocols.
- **Your local American Cancer Society chapter**

Is Hormone-Replacement Therapy Okay After Chemotherapy?

This is a very hot issue. Some say that because cancer cells feed on estrogen, why take more estrogen? Others believe hormone replacement after breast cancer can be safe if properly administered and after an appropriate time interval to be certain there has been no recurrence. Some believe progesterone-replacement therapy is okay because the risk is lower. Gynecologists, who administer hormone-replacement therapy, tend to be more positive about it for treatment of menopausal symptoms and for prevention of osteoporosis and cardiovascular problems. However, hormone-replacement therapy after breast cancer is generally discouraged by breast cancer physicians.

You need to discuss this at length with your gynecologist, medical oncologist, and surgeon. Also, ask what alternatives are available. How much estrogen is given to you depends upon the goal of treatment and whether or not your uterus is intact. There are alternatives for menopausal symptoms. Estrogen cream eases vaginal dryness (although it may be absorbed into the system in very small amounts). A glass of milk a day and weight-bearing exercise can help prevent osteoporosis. Diet and exercise can reduce the risk of cardiovascular disease. This is a very individual matter and needs careful consideration.

The Cost of Chemotherapy

What you pay for chemotherapy depends on what drugs you are getting, how much you are getting, and where you are getting your treatments. The cost of chemotherapy includes doctor visits and all the laboratory tests throughout your treatment, as well as other medications and a wig. All of this is generally included in health insurance coverage. If your insurance does not cover this, or if you have no insurance, some of the drug companies provide drugs for treatment. Your chemotherapist, the National Cancer Institute, or the local American Cancer Society chapter should have information about your area.

Tamoxifen is simply a bottle of pills (Nolvadex) that you refill as needed. A month's supply costs approximately $100; there is no cheaper version. If you are over fifty, check with the American Association of Retired Persons (AARP) prescription plan to see if you can get it cheaper. The company that manufactures the drug will sometimes provide it free to those unable to pay. You will probably be taking tamoxifen for five years or more, so it's a substantial investment.

Ask your chemotherapist to write for the *Directory of Prescription Drug Indigent Programs,* which can help locate drugs at low or no cost. This is published by the Pharmaceutical Manufacturers Association in Washington, D.C.

✔ Questions to Ask About Chemotherapy

These questions are meant to help you interview physicians and other healthcare professionals so that you can feel secure about your treatment decisions. Some of these questions have no clear-cut answers, some do. But ask anyway!

How do I know if I need cytotoxic drugs or tamoxifen?

You should find out your hormone-receptor status, tumor size, and lymph node status. These are probably the three most important factors in this decision. Expect your oncologist to go over all of this with you.

What is the goal of treatment?

This is important. Is the chemotherapy expected to cure you? Shrink your tumor before surgery? Control the spread of the disease? Prevent it from coming back?

How will the drug affect me? What are the side effects?

Your oncologist should explain how the drugs work in your body, and describe all the side effects you can expect.

Are there medications to counteract side effects?

Zofran helps stem nausea and vomiting. There are other drugs for this, as well as drugs to numb your mouth or throat and alleviate the pain of mouth sores.

How long will the treatments last?

Most cytotoxic chemotherapy is administered for three to six months before and/or after surgery. It used to be done for two to four years!

How will the medication be administered?

It can be oral or intravenous, depending upon your tolerance to the drugs and dose required. Some treatments require overnight hospitalization. A port may be implanted near your collarbone. Find out if your doctor or an assistant will be giving you your treatments.

Will chemotherapy affect my ability to have children?

Many women go through premature menopause after chemotherapy, and you need to know in advance if this may happen to you. If it isn't expected to force you into menopause, you still want to know how risky it will be to have children later. You need to consider the medical risks of pregnancy on your hormone levels and possibility of recurrence. There are numerous psychosocial issues to discuss if you've had cancer and elect to have children.

~ 9

Treatment for Advanced
Breast Cancer

The treatment of any advanced breast cancer requires focusing on the whole body, but the treatment is very different for locally advanced cancer, Stage III, and metastatic breast cancer, Stage IV. In treating locally advanced breast cancer, the goal is potential cure. Treatment for metastatic disease focuses on easing the symptoms and halting progression of the disease for as long as possible in order to maintain a decent quality of life.

Locally Advanced Breast Cancer

Treatment for locally advanced breast cancer has made great strides in recent years with the use of aggressive neoadjuvant, or induction, chemotherapy. If patients respond well to three to six months of chemotherapy, and their tumors shrink, they can have a mastectomy or even conserve their breast with lumpectomy, axillary dissection, and radiation. Then more chemotherapy is added to treatment for six to nine months.

Studies at several major medical centers of women with locally advanced breast cancer showed that two-year disease-free survival increased dramatically when they were given chemotherapy before surgery. The rate was 61 percent after five years and 55 percent after ten years. This study, one of the largest of its kind in this country, was conducted at Thomas Jefferson University in Philadelphia. Most of the women responded to the neoadjuvant chemotherapy with significant tumor regression. They could then be treated with mastectomy alone, or with lumpectomy and radiation followed by further chemotherapy.

If there is no response to chemotherapy, then radiation therapy can be an option, either by itself or with mastectomy.

Autologous Bone Marrow Transplantation

Chemotherapy and bone marrow transplantation is now offered to *cure* breast cancer. Its use is now being considered for premenopausal women with more than ten positive lymph nodes. Preliminary studies show it to work slightly better than conventional chemotherapy for locally advanced breast cancer.

Bone marrow is the red, pulpy substance inside your bones. It's where white cells, red cells, and platelets are produced before they are released into your bloodstream. Traditional bone marrow transplantation — from one person to another — has been in use since 1968, but one of the biggest difficulties is finding a donor match. Transplantation of marrow from another person also holds a higher risk of rejection or infection.

With autologous bone marrow transplantation (*autologous* means "from the same person"), some of the patient's own bone marrow is extracted, treated, and stored. This is a reserve supply. Chemotherapy is administered to the patient to destroy cancer cells in the remaining marrow and the rest of the body. Then the stored bone marrow is put back into the patient. This system requires no donor, and the risk of rejection or infection is reduced. A study at Duke University in the early 1990s showed a three-year disease-free survival of 72 percent in a group of eighty-five women with ten or more positive lymph nodes. A larger cooperative study is under way to confirm these findings.

Autologous bone marrow transplant can be performed only in a few specialized centers under protocol settings. This means everybody gets the same treatment and is followed up the same way. It is an expensive and prolonged procedure and requires a high level of skilled support services.

If bone marrow transplant is a treatment option, talk with your oncologist and call the bone marrow transplant program director where the treatment will take place. Find out how many breast cancer patients have been treated, the rate of cure and survival, and the cost of treatment. Ask about the clinical trials now in progress. You can get more information by calling the American Cancer Society (800-ACS-2345) and the bone marrow transplant resources listed later in this chapter.

How a Bone Marrow Transplant Is Performed

The procedure involves many people — physicians, facilitator nurse practitioners, social workers, psychologists, sometimes nutritionists, and biofeedback therapists. There must be lots of support and counseling for you and your family. It will take several months until it is completed.

First some of your bone marrow is removed and checked for cancer cells. Marrow is usually extracted from your pelvis; the pelvis is an excellent marrow producer and is close to the skin, making it easy to access the marrow through a syringe. The extracted marrow is stored for later use. Next, you get chemotherapy treatment. Then the stored bone marrow is returned to your body, and there is a period of several months until the marrow is functioning fully. You may spend part of the time in the hospital and part of the time as an outpatient.

Side effects of the treatment are similar to those of conventional chemotherapy, but may be more intense: nausea and vomiting, gastrointestinal discomfort, mouth sores, decreased white blood cells and platelets, and, potentially, damage to other organs. Because bone marrow has been destroyed by chemotherapy, infection is more common, and this can complicate the situation. Therefore, strict isolation precautions are followed, and antibiotics may be given to help prevent this.

Follow-up care is the same as with any chemotherapy treatment. Every few months you will see your doctor for a physical examination and blood tests.

The cost of autologous bone marrow transplantation, using outpatient procedures, is between $50,000 and $100,000.

To Find Out More About Bone Marrow Transplantation

There is a growing information network about bone marrow transplantation.

- **The BMT Newsletter**   708-831-1913
  This is a bimonthly publication with information from those who have had bone marrow transplant.
- **NABCO Hotline**   212-719-0154
  Ask for their information packet on bone marrow transplantation.
- **National Bone Marrow Transplant Link**   800-LINK-BMT
  This is an information clearinghouse and link with other patients and families of patients.
- **NCI Cancer Information Service**
  Hotline   800-4-CANCER
  Ask for information on clinical trials, and where to get treatment.

The Future of Bone Marrow Transplantation

A developing method of bone marrow transplantation lets doctors take bone marrow cells from a patient's *blood* for self-transplantation. These cells, called stem cells, mature more quickly than cells extracted from bone and help speed recovery. When treated with growth factors, stem cells multiply 1,000 times faster. Hospitalization is reduced from weeks to days. However, doctors must be able to ensure that those stem cells are viable, that they will proliferate and function. Once perfected, this process will offer a much less painful and difficult way to do bone marrow transplantation. Scientists hope to find a way to spur stem cell growth directly in the blood.

Treatment for Metastatic Breast Cancer

The goal of treatment for systemically advanced breast cancer is to create a balance whereby the disease is no longer spreading and thus no longer winning. Chemotherapy temporizes and palliates advanced disease. The aim is to control further spread for as long as possible. Some physicians use hormonal agents alone (tamoxifen, megestrol), others may use chemotherapy alone or chemotherapy and tamoxifen. It depends on where the disease is showing symptoms (this can be in the lungs, bones, liver, or brain) whether or not the tumor was hormone sensitive, and the time span between the first diagnosis and metastatic development.

Sometimes radiation may be necessary to palliate pain in the bone if chemotherapy is not working in certain spots. But radiation would be given locally, as spot treatment only. For example, if a tumor is obstructing a bronchial tube and causing breathing difficulty, then we can treat that small area with radiation to help relieve this. If there is compression on the spinal cord, a small radiation field can treat that, too.

New Treatments on the Horizon

Breast cancer research has accelerated since research funds finally became available. In fiscal 1993–94 federal funds for breast cancer research went from zero to $400 million as a result of intensive grassroots action by women all over the country. But we have a lot of catching up to do for all the years of neglect in breast cancer research. Research dollars are being used to advance our knowledge of breast cancer in relation to molecular genetics, drugs, nutrition, and environmental factors.

Molecular genetics. The BRCA1 gene has been identified in women from high-risk families. Eventually we hope to be able to test for this gene and use this information for counseling women and their families.

Another gene, the HER-2/neu gene, is abnormal in 30 percent of breast cancer patients. It is suspected that HER-2/neu is involved in producing protein receptors on the surface of breast cells. These receptors signal the cells to divide when growth factor molecules bind to them. Researchers are looking for an antibody that will fit the receptor to block it but will send no signal. Clinical trials with HER-2/neu began in 1993, with results expected around 1995. Many pathologists already test for the presence of HER-2/neu in breast cancer histologic studies, because it is a way to begin to see if it is a good prognostic factor.

Gene-replacement therapy. Once we identify the genes responsible for breast cancer, we hope to be able to screen patients to identify those at risk. Then we would be able to take a bad gene out of a person and replace it with a healthy one.

Breast cancer vaccine. In breast cancer cells, a protein known as breast epithelial mucin lacks part of its usual carbohydrate coating. Researchers are working to target this abnormal molecule. Mucin vaccine would stimulate the patient's own immune system to recognize and attack the abnormal molecules.

Diet. Many studies are focused on diet and breast cancer. See Chapter 15 to find out what's been discovered about what we eat.

✔ Questions to Ask About Treating Advanced Breast Cancer

These questions are meant to help you interview physicians and other healthcare professionals so that you can feel secure about your treatment decisions. Some of these questions have no clear-cut answers, some do. But ask anyway!

What stage is my cancer?

Locally advanced (Stage III) and systemically advanced (Stage IV) breast cancer are treated differently from each other and differently from Stage I and II cancers. You should also be aware that there is a difference between a cancer that was Stage III (locally advanced) at presentation and those smaller tumors with an earlier (lower) clinical stage that are upgraded to a more advanced stage by findings at the time of surgery, such as positive nodes. Staging can be more precisely defined using subdivisions such as Stage IIIA or IIB. Find out all the characteristics of your disease and its staging, so that you can more fully understand your treatment options, the goal of treatment, and the risks you are facing. It is important that you understand the histologic diagnosis — what your cells are showing — because it can affect the type of chemotherapy treatment you might receive and help determine the need for bone marrow transplantation.

What are my options for local and systemic treatment?

This is a multidisciplinary concern, so all of your treatment team should be involved with you in the decisions. Which area is most life threatening? That's where you start to concentrate. Your options depend on your particular situation, and treatment may include chemotherapy, surgery, radiation, and possibly bone marrow transplantation.

Can I have breast conservation treatment?

If your breast cancer is locally advanced and you respond well to neoadjuvant chemotherapy — that is, your tumor shrinks by more than 50 percent — it may be possible for you to have a lumpectomy and axillary dissection followed by radiation and chemotherapy. Each case is unique.

How will I be followed after all treatment is completed?

Be sure that all your follow-up care is explained. How often will you be examined and by whom? What studies or tests will need to be done periodically to monitor for response to treatment and watch for recurrence?

Is autologous bone marrow transplant an option for me?

This is something you must discuss carefully with your treatment team. If this course is an option for you, find out everything you can, including the latest information about the recommended transplant center. This procedure has been used successfully for breast cancer, but no long-term studies have been completed yet.

~ 10

Special Situations: When Other Medical Conditions or Pregnancy Must Be Considered

Sometimes concurrent or prior medical conditions can affect your breast cancer treatment, directly or indirectly. These are often conditions that would increase the risk of complications. Your family doctor or other medical specialist needs to be consulted by your breast cancer treatment team.

How Past and Present Medical Conditions Affect Treatment

Your treatment options may be limited by your previous medical history or a continuing condition. For instance, if you had cancer before, or radiation therapy, particularly to the chest or neck, you might not be able to have it again. Each area of your body has a limit to how much radiation it can tolerate. A similar cumulative effect can result from previous chemotherapy. Certain drugs would be unavailable to you the second time around.

With respect to ongoing conditions, a diabetic receiving chemotherapy, for example, could have a low blood sugar reaction if she is unable to maintain her proper diet. If she is using insulin, dosage may need to be adjusted. A woman with a heart condition would not be able to take some of the cytotoxic drugs, such as Adriamycin. A recent heart attack could also mean no general anesthesia could be given within three months of that attack. Obesity and cigarette smoking could also preclude general anesthesia. Someone with a collagen vascular disease, like scleroderma, would not be able to have radiation treatment because her skin would not tolerate it. She would not be able to tolerate reconstruction either.

Women who are housebound may not be able to get back and forth for radiation treatment. Because this must be done daily within the prescribed number of weeks, and radiation equipment cannot come to you, this could mean another treatment option must be planned.

If You Are Pregnant with Breast Cancer

Many women have healthy pregnancies after breast cancer. But when breast cancer is discovered during pregnancy, some very big issues have to be faced. Your wish to keep your baby must be weighed against possible harm to your baby and yourself if you get standard treatment — and if you don't.

Each woman comes with a different diagnosis — and a different set of values. If you decide to get an abortion, you don't have all these medical issues to worry about; but you have the emotional upheaval of losing the baby. Fortunately, fewer than 5 percent of breast cancer patients are pregnant at the time of diagnosis. We can't say how the prognosis looks because we haven't studied very many cases. It is possible that the chaotic state of hormones during pregnancy will feed the tumor and that it could even regress somewhat after a therapeutic abortion. But we don't know for sure. Women who are diagnosed later in the pregnancy usually have normal pregnancies and healthy babies.

Five years ago, a thirty-nine-year-old patient who discov-

ered a mass as a hard spot in her breast six weeks before her
baby was due had a mastectomy and delivered a healthy baby
on schedule. She had a 1-centimeter mass and negative lymph
nodes. Had she not been pregnant, she would probably have
had lumpectomy and radiation. She ultimately had a delayed
reconstruction using a tissue-expander.

Breasts are even more lumpy when you are pregnant, and
women often don't do their breast self-examination (BSE),
and so breast cancer is frequently more advanced by the time
it's discovered. Remember, if you notice a change, or mass,
even while you are pregnant or nursing, bring it to the attention of your physician immediately so it can be evaluated with
ultrasound, needle cytology, or surgical biopsy with local anesthesia. Mammogram can be used but may be limited. Treatment depends on which trimester you are in when the breast
cancer diagnosis is made, as well as the answers to these
questions:

- What would be the best treatment if I were not pregnant?
- How will my treatment be compromised by the pregnancy?
- What is the risk of treatment to the baby?

Treatment of Early Breast Cancer

If you were not pregnant, you might be treated with lumpectomy followed by radiation. But if you are in your first trimester of pregnancy, when the baby's organs are being formed,
radiation or chemotherapy is risky.

If you want to keep the baby, you may need to make some
compromises in your treatment options. Mastectomy is a way
to avoid radiation exposure to the baby. Or you may have to
delay your workup and treatment until later in the pregnancy,
or even after delivery, and be willing to accept the potential
compromise to your health.

Avoiding Some of the Risks of Radiation

Radiation exposure at an early stage of fetal development (first trimester), from a routine X-ray workup or from treatment, can lead to malformations. Radiation exposure in the second or third trimester can lead to growth retardation, behavioral abnormalities, and potential tumors. You must be informed of all the risks to the fetus from X-ray studies such as mammograms, bone scans, and CAT scans. Ask for a lead shield to cover your abdomen during any radiation exposure.

Blood tests. To check for metastasis, some blood tests can be done instead of a bone scan, which would expose the fetus to about 100 mrads of radiation. (An mrad, or millirad, is 0.001 rad.) If these tests show no metastasis you can do without a bone scan or at least wait until after you have delivered.

Ultrasound can be used to look at your affected breast if you are getting a mastectomy. However, you still need a mammogram of the opposite breast to be certain the cancer is not bilateral.

A surgical biopsy under local anesthesia is okay, with minimal risk to the fetus. Because your breast is engorged during pregnancy, there is more bleeding with surgery, but this is manageable.

If Radiation Therapy Must Be Done

No matter how sophisticated the radiation treatment facility, there is always what is called internal scatter. The photons or X rays may bounce off tissues in the breast and scatter elsewhere inside the patient. Scatter is of no consequence to a mature woman, but to a developing fetus it's dangerous. To accommodate the pregnancy, radiation therapy could be done in reverse order, with the boost first. This focuses an intense dose on the tumor site and is normally done after the weeks of radiation to the entire breast. Treatment to the whole breast could be postponed until the fetus is more mature. You could delay radiation until after delivery, but waiting more than eight to twelve weeks after a lumpectomy to start radiation therapy increases chances of local recurrence.

The Risks of Anesthesia and Surgery

Choosing a mastectomy rather than lumpectomy for early breast cancer is one way to avoid the dangers of radiation, but you still face the risks of general anesthesia. In the first trimester of pregnancy it could precipitate premature labor and spontaneous abortion. If you can wait until the second trimester of pregnancy, that risk is very low, probably less than 2 percent. In the later stages of pregnancy, this is not much of a problem, since organ development is established and the placenta is developed. By the third trimester, the baby is more self-sufficient and likely to survive even with premature labor.

Pregnancy and More Advanced Breast Cancer

You may be able to get by without a full staging workup with early breast cancer, but if your cancer is advanced, you really need a full workup to find out if it has spread. You need to be fully informed about the risks to the fetus from the X rays you must have to rule out metastatic disease. If you are in your first trimester, most physicians would recommend abortion. If you are too far into the pregnancy to have an abortion, then chemotherapy may have to be a consideration without delay — despite the potential risk to your child. If you are at the end stages of pregnancy, chemotherapy, which would be a major part of your treatment, can be delayed until after delivery.

Why is chemotherapy a problem during pregnancy? Chemotherapy is a systemic treatment. It goes everywhere in your body. This is very good when you are trying to kill cancer cells, but you will also be giving the medication to your baby. And your baby will suffer the side effects with you. Some drugs do not cross the placental barrier, but there are other repercussions. If the drugs can make you sick, cause you to become dehydrated, or not eat the balanced diet that is vital to your baby's growth and development, then your baby is in jeopardy. You should not underestimate the potential complications of chemotherapy during pregnancy. The risk for fetal malformations is greatest during the first trimester. There is no reported risk of malformation during the second or third trimesters, but there are very few patients to study in this category. Spontaneous abortion is also a risk in the first trimester. The risk of your child developing solid tumors and leukemias later on in childhood is unknown but must be considered. Because there have been more of these kinds of tumors in patients treated with chemotherapy, investigators are questioning whether it is caused by treatment or is a predisposition given the family history of cancer.

Having breast cancer is an emotional jolt and so is being pregnant. Experiencing both at the same time is a double whammy, and you need a good support system around you to keep from being overwhelmed. You do have options, and you have to give them all careful consideration.

~ 11

Support Groups: Part of the Treatment, Part of the Cure

The initial response to the breast cancer diagnosis is disbelief and shock. It is perfectly normal to be afraid and anxious. This is extremely depressing news, after all, and you may have all sorts of preconceived notions about what is going to happen to you. Many women ask, Why me? What did I do? How could I have avoided this? Don't blame yourself. It won't help you recover. *You did not give yourself breast cancer.* We don't yet know what causes breast cancer, but we do know that in some cases it is genetic. We also know that breast cancer support groups work. Not only do women participating in support groups survive longer, they are less anxious, less depressed, less afraid, and experience less pain. We are active in these groups ourselves, and always recommend them, because we know they offer one of the best ways to get yourself through a rough time. There is a wonderful warmth and camaraderie in a group of women who have survived breast cancer. It's a place where you can feel safe and secure. Here, everybody understands and you do not have to hide your fears, or pretend everything is all right. There is room and caring to express your anger, shed your tears, and get a hug.

Why Support Groups Work

Some women look for a support group as soon as they get the diagnosis; others seek one out after treatment, or after recurrence. Some don't go until someone close to them develops breast cancer. Go now. This is not the time to hide away by yourself. Even a loving family and friends are not enough. You need to talk with other women who know what it's like to have breast cancer. It's important to see for yourself that there is life after breast cancer — a good life. If you are coping, you may also be a role model for another woman.

The weeks and months after diagnosis are fraught with anxiety, as the staging procedures, blood tests, and scans are happening; as surgery, chemotherapy, or radiation is anticipated. As you become more familiar with the treatment routine, your anxiety will diminish. Nevertheless, the diagnosis and treatment can compromise your self-esteem and sexuality, and it can disrupt your family and schedule.

Support groups help you through this, by letting you know how others cope with their jobs, changing family roles, household responsibilities, family resentments, children's fears, friends who don't know what to say or do. This is a lot for you to worry about on top of worrying about breast cancer. You don't have to prove how brave you are. Don't do it alone! There is no substitute for the emotional bond that develops among women in a breast cancer support group. There are support groups for spouses and families, too.

One woman who knew nothing about breast cancer sought out a support group as soon as she was diagnosed — just to be there and find out what she could. When asked her biggest fear, she said, "I'm afraid they'll find cancer everywhere." She said her life had been filled with struggle and she didn't think she could get through yet another one, which could be a long and stressful cancer treatment. The others had the same fears. They told her what chemotherapy and radiation and surgery felt like. They shared their own personal stories and methods of getting through it. They laughed and joked about wigs and weight gain or loss, and talked about how their lives had changed — how they were learning how to live, really live.

At the next meeting, the group asked the new patient how she felt. Still terrified, she did manage a smile and said, "Well, I've decided to live." The others cheered loudly and gave her a standing ovation. One of them sent her a greeting card every day for the first month, just to let her know she was not alone.

How to Find a Support Group

It would be unusual if you could not find a breast cancer support group in your community. There are well over three hundred from coast to coast, and more are forming every day. In addition, almost every hospital has one. If there are no support groups in your area, think about starting one. This takes a lot of work but may be rewarding. To find one near you, ask at your hospital social work department, or call the following:

- **American Cancer Society**   800-ACS-2345
  Call to find out how to get in touch with your local chapter.
- **NABCO Hotline**   212-719-0154
  The resource booklet ($3) lists all the known breast cancer support groups in the country.
- **Y-ME National Hotline**   800-221-2141
  They have chapters in many states and Canada and will help you start a support group.
- **Your local YWCA**
  Ask about the ENCORE program for postoperative breast cancer patients.

Private Counseling

If you are unable to participate in a support group, you may want to talk with a psychologist or psychiatrist — preferably a woman — for short-term support. There is a newly developing therapeutic specialty called psycho-oncology, and you may be able to locate a therapist who specializes in the emotional aspects of cancer. More often than not, short-term counseling once or twice a week is all that is needed to get you through the treatment process. Therapy can be one-on-one or with your family. Some of these resources may be able to help you locate someone:

- your local hospital oncology or psychiatry department
- the American Medical Association
- the American Psychiatric Association

Using Biofeedback to Reduce Stress

Some cancer centers may offer behavioral therapy such as visualization, biofeedback, and relaxation techniques, which help you cope and feel in control of your treatment and recovery. Biofeedback is a technique of learning to monitor some of your own involuntary processes and then intervene to modify them. Skin electrodes monitor subtle changes in temperature, muscle tension, perspiration, blood pressure, and heart rate and rhythm. By observing what your body is doing — signals from the electrodes form graphs on a video screen — you can learn to intervene. Patients have learned to reduce blood pressure, relax muscle tension, and control pain.

Women who have excessive discomfort after mastectomy and lymph node dissection or who are afraid to use their arm, have learned to increase mobility and strength with biofeedback. It can also help you relax before treatments and reduce the symptoms of nausea and vomiting caused by chemotherapy.

Most large hospital psychiatry departments and an increasing number of cancer centers have a biofeedback therapist on staff. Medical insurance often covers this therapy. Take advantage of everything that is available to you. This is your time to take care of you.

~ **III**

Recovery:
What to Expect After
Treatment

~ 12

Who's in Charge of Your Follow-up Care?

Your surgeon, plastic surgeon, radiation oncologist, and medical oncologist monitor your healing process periodically and check for possible recurrence. In addition to careful physical examinations every three to four months, you need a mammogram every six months for two years, blood tests if you are taking cytotoxic drugs or tamoxifen, and possibly a bone scan or other screenings depending on your situation.

Who is going to coordinate all of this? Your gynecologist is rarely involved as the coordinator after initial screening, although regular gynecological checkups are now mandatory. Often your surgeon, the first doctor who treated you, coordinates your follow-up care. If you feel most comfortable with your family doctor, then ask if he or she will coordinate your care. But whether or not any of your doctors agrees to be an overseer, your follow-up care won't get organized, and appointments won't get made, unless you are in charge. It's up to you to keep each of your doctors informed about what the others are doing.

Setting Up a Schedule

Try to schedule your appointments with your surgeon, radiologist, and oncologist so your breasts, lymph nodes, and vital signs are being examined by one of them at least every three months for the first two years. If you see everyone during the same day or week, then months can go by without an exam that could pick up a possible recurrence. Keep track of your visits and schedules in an appointment book and know when your next examination is due. Do this in a routine, businesslike way and it will be easier to handle. You will always feel anxious before your next mammogram or bone scan. Everyone does. But don't let anxiety prevent you from doing it. Here is a summary of procedures you will need during the next two to five years and a roster of the doctors you should see.

BSE. The monthly breast self-examination is the most important part of your vigilance. Most breast cancers are found this way. There is more about this later in the chapter. You are not looking for cancer, you are looking for change. If change occurs, bring it directly to a physician's attention.

Mammogram. If you had a lumpectomy, you need a mammogram every six months for two years on the treated breast, and yearly on the opposite breast. After that, once a year is generally enough. Radiologists will be particularly watchful when they look at your films now, and they may want to take additional pictures, or may make you wait longer while your films are studied. This will make you tense, but it's always best to get a thorough reading of your film. If you had a mastectomy, then your remaining breast needs to be X-rayed annually unless there is an abnormality that warrants evaluation. A mammogram is not necessary for a reconstructed breast.

Surgeon. If you had a mastectomy, your surgeon will examine your chest wall to be sure you are healing properly and you are not developing a seroma (fluid under the skin) or flap necrosis (when the skin at the wound edges dies), a rare occurrence. Your opposite breast and all the lymph node areas should be examined every two to four weeks until you are healed and then every three months. If you had a lumpectomy, your surgeon sees you every three or six months for the first two years. If you had an axillary dissection, your surgeon may measure your arm if you have any evidence or complaints of lymphedema (swelling), and ascertain whether you have full range of motion in your arm.

Plastic surgeon. Because reconstruction is a complex and sometimes lengthy procedure, visits to your plastic surgeon will be frequent — every two weeks or so — following surgery. This surgeon must evaluate symmetry, implant integrity, mobility, and your satisfaction, in addition to checking for wound healing and signs of infection, and doing additional procedures, such as nipple reconstruction.

Radiation oncologist. If you had chest wall or breast radiation therapy, your radiation oncologist will examine you every six months for any lingering redness or swelling and to monitor for recurrence. This doctor will review your mammography reports, measure your arm for signs of swelling — either from radiation or the axillary dissection — and photograph your breast to record your healing progress. Try to coordinate your visit so that you have your mammogram before visiting your radiation oncologist.

Medical oncologist. If you are receiving cytotoxic chemotherapy, your oncologist will routinely monitor your blood before and during treatment and then yearly. Your oncologist examines you for evidence of recurrence (particularly in the node-bearing areas and liver and lungs) and asks if you have any complaints about side effects. If you are taking tamoxifen, your oncologist performs a general physical examination, including a breast exam, every three months for the first two years, then every six months. Your blood is analyzed for evidence of metastatic disease and also to indicate how the medication is affecting you. Once treatment is over and your white blood cells and platelets are stable, yearly blood counts are all that is necessary to monitor for metastasis.

If you have invasive breast cancer a bone scan should be done annually. Some oncologists may not want to order this test for you if your risk of metastasis is very low, because it's an expensive test. The likelihood of testing positive in the absence of symptoms, such as bone pain, is very low (1–2 percent).

Gynecologist. In addition to a routine gynecological examination and Pap test, your other concerns may include birth control or menopausal symptoms. If you are premenopausal you cannot use birth control pills, especially if you take tamoxifen. If you are postmenopausal and have menopausal symptoms, you may want to discuss alternatives to hormone-replacement therapy. For instance, there are a variety of lubricants available for vaginal dryness. Estrogen replacement is generally not advised after breast cancer.

Family doctor. While other physicians are keeping tabs on your breast cancer, your overall health needs attention. An annual physical checkup should be part of your routine. You absolutely need an annual chest X ray to monitor your lungs for signs of cancer; other tests and lab work depend on your age and condition. If you are over fifty, have a colonoscopy every year or two. This aids in early detection for colon cancer, and once you've had any cancer you are at increased risk. Keep your family doctor well informed about your follow-up care with specialists.

Ophthalmologist. Let your ophthalmologist know if you are taking tamoxifen, and have your eyes checked annually. In very rare cases, tamoxifen can affect your vision.

How to Do Your Monthly Breast Self-exam

From now on, this is the most crucial part of your follow-up care. Get to know your breasts intimately — how they look and how they feel inside and out. Your own examination is very effective and accurate and more frequent than an exam by a physician, who is not familiar with *your* breasts. More than half of all breast cancers are found this way. It's not difficult, and all we ask is that you look for *change* — anything that is different about your breasts, such as swelling, skin rash, discoloration, puckering, an area of thickening, or discharge from the nipple. Bring it to someone's attention for further evaluation.

If you are premenopausal, the ideal time for your breast self-exam is one week after the first day of your period. Otherwise, your breasts are influenced by hormones and may be too lumpy. If you are postmenopausal, pick a day each month and always do your BSE on that date. If you have never done a BSE before, make an appointment with your surgeon or radiation or medical oncologist to learn the technique and some basic breast anatomy. Some physicians have plastic breast forms implanted with small pellets so that you can learn what to look for.

Pregnant or nursing women should continue to do BSE despite the lumpiness that can accompany these conditions. You know your breasts well and you can still find a lump when it is small.

Do your BSE standing up and lying down. The shower is convenient because your hand glides over lathered skin easily. The top half of the breast is easy to examine when standing because gravity pulls the weight of the breast down. But first, make a visual inspection. Stand facing a mirror with your hands on your hips and look at your breasts. Do they look different in any way? Bend forward and look again. Then raise your arms over your head and look. Turn to each side and look. Squeeze your nipples to see if fluid can be expressed.

When lying down, push a pillow under your shoulder and raise your arm over your head. Use the pads of three fingers of your opposite hand to palpate your breast. Don't forget about the tail of your breast, which goes up into the axilla. There are three patterns of palpation: circular, vertical, or radial. Choose the method that works for you and do it consistently so you become very familiar with how your breasts look and feel.

• Circular method: Start at your nipple and palpate in a clockwise direction around your breast with progressively larger circles.

• Vertical method: Palpate up and down your breast from your collarbone to your ribs, working from the center of your chest out to your underarm.

• Radial, or "pie," method: Mentally divide your breast into wedges. Start at the outside edge of the breast and work your way in to the nipple, palpating one wedge at a time. Start superficially, then press deeper, to the chest wall.

Free BSE guides — including videos — are available in English and Spanish from a variety of sources, including most hospitals. Ask your doctors or check with either of these agencies:

• **American Cancer Society**   800-ACS-2345
They have a waterproof shower card with illustrated instructions.

• **NCI Cancer Information Service**
Hotline   800-4-CANCER
An illustrated instruction booklet with poster is available.

Many private agencies, such as the Avon Foundation and the Liz Claiborne Foundation, offer BSE materials.

✔ Questions to Ask About Follow-up Care

These questions are meant to help you interview physicians and other healthcare professionals so that you can feel secure about your treatment decisions. Some of these questions have no clear-cut answers, some do. But ask anyway!

How should I coordinate my follow-up care with you and my other doctors?

All of your doctors should pay attention and respond to this. Some are more willing than others to think about your overall situation. Some may only want to handle whatever they are treating, like your chemotherapy, and let you handle the rest. Be sure each one has clearly outlined his or her follow-up program.

How will you communicate information to my other doctors?

If all of your doctors are in the same medical center, it will be fairly easy to access your medical records. But paper moves slowly in any large organization. Ask how your oncologist will transmit information to your surgeon — phone, fax, mail — if there is a need for them to confer about a symptom, such as a swelling, which could be a result of surgery or radiation.

To whom should my mammogram report be sent?

The doctor who prescribed the mammogram will usually get the report, unless he or she specifically directs that it be sent to another. All of your cancer doctors should get a copy — surgeon, medical and radiation oncologists, as well as your gynecologist and family doctor.

Who will decide if I need a periodic bone scan or other screening for metastasis?

If you have invasive cancer, even with a very slim chance of recurrence, most doctors are willing to do a bone scan if you request it. Talk with your medical oncologist about doing this annually. If you have more advanced breast cancer you *must* have this done, and your oncologist will probably prescribe this for you.

Should I have periodic blood tests to check for bone and liver metastasis?

This is routine and is usually done annually by your medical oncologist. In addition to tumor markers, there are special studies, such as alkaline phosphatase for bone metastasis. These, and others such as the liver enzymes (GGTP, SGOT, SGPT), check for liver metastasis.

What symptoms should I check for or try to be aware of?

Your doctor should explain the kinds of things to be aware of, such as persistent bone pain, or pain that increases in severity, headaches, blurred vision, fever, or any signal from your body that seems unusual. Bring any new complaint to the attention of one of your doctors.

Whom do I call if I have any of these symptoms?

Call your medical oncologist if you are on chemotherapy, otherwise talk with your family doctor first if you like. But never hesitate to call any of the physicians on your treatment team.

How can I learn BSE?

Your doctors and nurses can review this procedure with you. There are also many pamphlets and videos available through the breast cancer support networks.

How often should I have a chest X ray?

You should have a chest X ray every year — not only to be sure your lungs are healthy, but to monitor for metastasis.

What other routine tests should I have now that I have had cancer?

In addition to your mammogram, you should have an annual gynecological checkup, a colonoscopy, and a general physical examination.

~ 13

Will You Get It Again?

Nobody knows if a cancer will recur. We can only calculate the odds based on everything we learn through diagnosis and treatment. By understanding type and size of tumor, cell activity, lymph node status, and staging, we can *estimate* that someone has a 10 percent chance of recurrence or a 65 percent chance, but this does not mean it *will* recur. Nor is there any guarantee that you *won't* have a recurrence even with a 5 percent chance.

Your breast cancer could recur in the same breast, the other breast, or elsewhere in your system, a year or decades later. Generally, five cancer-free years means you've beaten the heaviest odds. Eighty percent of recurrences happen within the first five years after initial treatment; 20 percent, years later. Breast cancer is very unpredictable. This is why frequent breast self-exams and follow-up care are so critical during the first five years after treatment. Recurrence can be:

- local — reappearance at the same site (the breast)
- regional — reappearance near the original site (lymph nodes)
- metastatic — reappearance elsewhere in your body (liver, lungs, bone, brain)

If you had an in situ ductal carcinoma, smaller than 1 centimeter (⅓ inch), with the least aggressive cells, you have the lowest chance of recurrence, often less than 5 percent. If you had a larger and invasive tumor with aggressive cells, and positive lymph nodes, then your risk of recurrence is higher, at least 30 percent. Your pathology reports can help you understand this. Many reports summarize these findings. Go over these reports with your doctors so you understand the information.

Understanding Unavoidable Risk Factors

A family history of breast cancer is a known risk factor, but only 15 to 20 percent of women who get breast cancer have that history. It is now believed that inherited breast cancer involves a faulty gene that has been named BRCA1 — for breast cancer 1. This gene is passed on through men and women in some families. It is estimated that a woman born to a carrier of the gene has a greater than 50 percent chance of getting breast cancer. A blood test will soon enable women from breast cancer families to find out their own risk. However, even if a woman did not inherit the BRCA1 gene, she is still at risk for getting nonhereditary breast cancer

Breast cancer seems to be a complex combination of genetics, hormones, diet, and environment. We don't know the cause yet, but at last there is more research in progress. With discovery and understanding of the genes involved, we will find better treatment and, ultimately, prevention, perhaps through gene therapy or vaccination. If you and the women in your family are at high risk, then be ever vigilant. Some women from high-risk families have had prophylactic mastectomy — removing both breasts so they cannot get breast cancer.

When the tamoxifen trial is completed in 1998 we should know more about the use of prophylactic tamoxifen to prevent breast cancer in women at high risk. In the meantime, be candid with your family members. They should be well informed about your breast cancer so they can understand their own risk. Women are genuinely concerned about risks their daughters and granddaughters face in the future. The National High-Risk Registry at the Strang Cancer Prevention Center in New York (800-921-9356) is one of the largest registries of women at high risk. The registry provides access to genetic counseling, a surveillance program, risk assessment, and other resources. The registry is affiliated with the New York Hospital–Cornell Medical Center.

Risk Factors You Can Avoid

You can't do much about genetic risk factors, but you are *absolutely* able to avoid risk factors like smoking, poor diet, lack of exercise, and exposure to known carcinogens in your environment. Just because you have breast cancer doesn't mean you cannot get other cancers, so avoid as many risk factors as you can. Your doctors should know if your lifestyle in any way contributes to your risk of recurrence, and help you to eliminate those risks.

Smoking. We know smoking causes lung, mouth, head, and neck cancer, as well as heart attacks and strokes. It is also being studied for its implication in breast cancer, but whether or not it is a direct cause, it is possibly an indirect one. Smoking is so bad for you that women who smoke may have more difficulty with general anesthesia and will usually be declined for free-flap breast reconstruction. Smoking causes vasospasm (spasm of the blood vessels), which can jeopardize the flap.

Improper Diet. According to the National Cancer Institute, one-third of all cancers are related to diet — primarily diets low in fiber and high in fat. Too much fat creates a climate conducive to cancer. Estrogen is stored in fat cells, and estrogen feeds cancer cells. Lack of fiber is a leading cause of colon cancer and may also be implicated in the production of a form of estrogen found in tumor tissue. There is more about diet in Chapter 15.

Alcohol. While scientists are debating whether alcohol is good or bad for our health, keep in mind that alcohol does interact with estrogen in a negative way. Studies show that while two drinks a day may lower your risk of heart disease, your risk for breast cancer is increased. If you are eating right and exercising regularly, your heart won't need alcohol. If you choose to drink, moderation is always wise.

Lack of exercise. Exercise affects your hormonal balance as well as most of your body's other systems. Athletes often have higher levels of the inert type of estrogen that protects from breast cancer, as opposed to the active type of estrogen found in breast cancer cells.

Estrogen-replacement therapy. We feel that estrogen increases the rate of recurrence in the breast cancer patient, but we don't know by how much. Estrogen-replacement therapy after menopause may or may not pose a risk for development of breast cancer, but most breast cancer doctors are uncomfortable using it after women have been treated for breast cancer. However, there is no standard thinking yet in the medical community. It is an individual decision that requires lengthy discussion and consideration of other problems, like osteoporosis or hot flashes. The pros and cons need a thoughtful and comprehensive assessment.

Radiation. Because you will need to be screened for recurrence, you may have more mammograms and possibly other X rays than if you had not had breast cancer. There is little danger from exposure to diagnostic radiation, but if you are in childbearing years, you may feel more secure covering your abdomen with a lead shield to protect your ovaries from radiation.

Watching for Signs of Recurrence

With regular follow-up care and your monthly BSE, you are maintaining vigilance. Try not to become obsessed with looking for a new cancer, but do pay attention to signals from your body, especially back and bone pain. Most bone metastases occur in the spine and the long bones of the arm and leg. Call your doctor if you have any symptoms like these:

- changes in the appearance of your breast; or redness, swelling, lumps, or thickening in your scar; or a rash on your chest
- persistent pain in your breast, shoulder, pelvis, lower back
- persistent coughing or hoarseness
- nausea, vomiting, diarrhea, or heartburn that lasts for several days
- loss of appetite or unexplained weight changes
- changes in your menstrual cycle or flow, or interval spotting
- dizziness, blurred vision, severe or frequent headaches, or trouble walking
- jaundice
- leg weakness, sciatica

Don't hesitate to bring anything new or persistent to your doctor's attention, especially if it intensifies. That's what we are here for. If it's of concern, we will pursue it. If it turns out not to be important, you will feel better.

✔ Questions to Ask About Breast Cancer
   Recurrence

*These questions are meant to help you interview physicians and
other healthcare professionals so that you can feel secure about your
treatment decisions. Some of these questions have no clear-cut
answers, some do. But ask anyway!*

**How can I understand chances of a recurrence of my breast
cancer?**

Your surgeon — and your other doctors, too — should truth-
fully explain your chances of recurrence based on how you
have responded to treatment and what your pathology report
indicates. If you feel the answer is vague, ask specific questions
about the information in your pathology report, but try not to
become fixated upon every detail of your breast cancer.

**What tests should I have to watch for local and systemic recur-
rence?**

In addition to BSE, mammography is a must to screen for local
recurrence. An annual chest X ray and periodic blood tests
can look for metastasis in the liver or bone. Bone scans can
also do this, but doctors often don't prescribe them if the risk
of recurrence is low. If you have invasive breast cancer, you
will want to know if you need an annual bone scan.

What is my risk of another primary in my other breast?

About 15–20 percent of patients will develop a new primary
in the other breast, about 1 percent a year. If you come from
a high-risk family, talk with your doctor about how the breast
cancer gene is inherited and passed on, and your own and your
children's chances of developing breast cancer. Ask about the
breast cancer high-risk registry. Most cities have such registries
at one or more medical centers to track the course of patients
and their families.

What risk factors can I avoid?

Your doctor should strongly urge you to change any bad habits, such as smoking, lack of exercise, and poor nutrition, that may contribute to your risk for recurrence or diminish your general health.

What treatment can I expect for a recurrence?

Treatment is constantly improving and may be different at the time of a possible recurrence. Treatment will also depend upon whether or not it's a local recurrence or a metastasis. Local recurrence could mean a re-excision or mastectomy. Regional (in the nodes) could mean mastectomy and/or chemotherapy with a lymph node dissection. Distant metastasis usually means chemotherapy, bone marrow transplant, or radiation or, less commonly, local surgery.

~ 14

A Primer on Lymphedema

Lymphedema happens. There seems no clear reason why some women are plagued by it and others are not. There has been very little scientific research about lymphedema after breast surgery and axillary dissection. Patients are rarely given good information about prevention and what to do if it occurs. Women are often told to restrict activity, when in fact activity and exercise are probably the best ways to prevent lymphedema and control it when it occurs.

Lymphedema is swelling caused by the inability of lymphatic fluid to circulate normally in your arm because some or all of your lymph nodes have been removed. It can become chronic if it is ignored. When lymph nodes are removed from the axilla, it's more difficult for the remaining nodes to handle all the traffic through the lymphatic vessels. It's like gridlock. Fluid may slow down until alternate channels are created, and this causes swelling. This backup of lymphatic fluid, rich in albumin (protein), creates a perfect environment for bacteria to grow.

Lymphedema can occur all by itself, or it can be brought about if you injure your arm or get an infection from a cut or scratch. Any injury causes lymphatic fluid to rush to the affected area to fight off inflammation. If the fluid doesn't find a way out, you have lymphedema. Your arm can be fine for years, and then one day something as seemingly inconsequential as a paper cut could cause it to swell up.

How to Know You Have It: Self-screening

If you know the normal circumference of your arm, you will be able to watch for lymphedema and treat it before it gets out of control. Your involved arm may always be half an inch larger than the other, and this is considered normal. Your surgeon or radiation therapist will have measured the circumference of your upper and lower arms — both the involved and uninvolved arm — before treatment to get a baseline measurement from which to gauge any change.

If they did not do this, then measure both arms now with a tape measure. This is not an exact method and does not replace a physician's checkup, but it gives you a baseline. Your bones — wrist and elbow — provide a point of reference. Measure the circumference of your arm six inches above your elbow crease, at the elbow crease, six inches below it, and just above your wrist. Don't pull the tape tightly, just circle your arm with it. It's easier to have someone else do it, but you can manage it alone by holding the tape with your arm close to your side. Take measurements before you go to bed and when you wake up. Your arm may be bigger at the end of the day and therefore may not provide a true indicator. Generally, a more than ½-inch difference from the normal circumference is considered swollen enough to do something about.

Postoperative Exercises to Help Prevent Lymphedema

One way to help prevent lymphedema is to keep your muscles loose and your lymphatic fluids circulating. Special exercises can begin a day or two after surgery, even with your drains still in place, but check with your doctor first. If your surgeon wants you to wait until the drains are out, then it may be a week before you begin your exercises. Sometimes the hospital physical therapist can work with you for the first few days.

Your surgery affected the muscles and nerves of your chest and arm as well as your lymph system. You need to exercise after surgery so your range of motion will not be limited. If you are to begin radiation therapy, you absolutely must exercise your arm three times a day so you can get it up over your head before treatment begins. If you can't move it, then part of your arm will be radiated along with your breast. If your arm is restricted at the start of radiation therapy and loosens up a week or two into treatments, your treatment may need to be replanned. A more relaxed arm later can cause a change in the radiation field. However, everyone is unique and some women have no trouble raising their arm. Others find it easy to raise their arm after surgery, then are shocked when a week later their arm tightens up. This is because the scar tissue is forming.

Range-of-Motion Exercises

Exercise three times a day, and do each exercise ten times. Exercise slowly, and don't bounce or jerk your arm. The slow stretch is the most effective and least likely to cause injury or strain. Your surgeon may have additional exercises for you to do. Some discomfort is normal right after surgery, but these exercises should not cause pain. If they do, stop and discuss it with your doctor.

Exercise 1. Stand up straight with your arms at your sides and your feet 12 inches apart. Bend forward from the waist so that your arms hang loosely in front of you. You may want to lean on something like a table or chair to support your back. Swing your affected arm like a pendulum in a wide clockwise circle ten times, then counterclockwise ten times. This will warm up your muscles.

Exercise 2. This is a bit more difficult. Stand straight with your feet together. Raise your affected arm sideways and put the palm of your hand on the back of your head. Bring your elbow forward and back, like flapping a wing. Do this ten times.

Exercise 3. Stand sideways at arm's length from a wall with your involved arm and shoulder facing the wall. Put your arm out to the side. "Walk" up the wall with your fingers, as high as you can. Do this ten times. Each time try to reach a little higher. It may be helpful to put a little mark on the wall so you can reach higher the next time. It is normal to feel your muscles pulling, but stop if you feel pain. Repeat this exercise facing the wall, with your arm straight out in front of you.

Exercise 4. Stand straight with your feet together. Place the fingers of your involved hand near your ear on the same side. Walk these fingers across the top of your head to the other ear. Don't bend your head toward your shoulder; that's cheating. Do this ten times.

The Importance of Exercise in Managing Lymphedema

Once you've done these exercises to gain your range of motion, begin exercises designed for flexibility and strength in your shoulder and arm. These are fairly simple and not at all time-consuming. Do them every day for the first year. It takes that long for scar tissue to finish growing. You need strength in your arms. When your arm muscles are weak, an injury is more likely to hurt you and cause the lymph fluid to fill up your arm.

In the past, women were told that any traction-type force, such as pushing (push-ups) or carrying a hanging weight, like a suitcase, was harmful, but there is no research to back this up. We urge our patients to do whatever they did before, as long as it doesn't hurt. Stretching and strengthening your muscles will keep you fit and help lymph fluid flow through your arm. An illustrated booklet of exercises designed for the management of lymphedema is available from the Breast Cancer Physical Therapy Center (see Appendix 4). Physical therapist Linda Miller, who wrote the booklet, gave us permission to share the following flexibility exercises with you here.

Flexibility Exercises

Stretching exercises for the axillary area and chest wall are extremely important. Tight muscles in this area can further complicate the problem by congesting the remaining nodes. Stretches are more effective if held for at least fifteen seconds. It is better to do fewer stretches for a longer duration. Don't bounce when stretching; hold a static stretch. A stretch should be "strainful" but never painful. Repeat all of these exercises ten times.

1. **Passive shoulder flexion.** This stretches the axilla and the muscles in the back of your arm. When you perform this exercise correctly, you feel a stretch in the axilla and along the back of your arm from shoulder to elbow. Stand facing a wall, an arm's length away, with your arm reaching up the wall as high as possible. Lean forward, move closer to the wall, and continue to reach until you feel a stretch in the axilla. Hold it for fifteen seconds. As your motion improves, begin the stretch standing farther away from the wall to increase the stretch.

2. **Assisted shoulder flexion.** This exercise stretches your axilla and the muscles in the back of your arm. It requires a wand or a lightweight stick about 18 inches long. Lie on your back on a firm surface. Hold the wand in front of you with your arms shoulder width apart, elbows straight. Raise the wand up over your head, keeping your elbows straight. Let the weight of your arms stretch out the axilla. Relax with the wand in this position. Hold for fifteen seconds. Slowly return to starting position. Don't allow your back to arch as you perform this

exercise. This will cause you to substitute back motion for arm motion and the stretch will be less effective.

3. **Assisted shoulder abduction.** This exercise stretches your axilla and the muscles on the inside of your arm and along the side of your body. When you do this correctly, you feel a stretch under your arm that may extend to the elbow. You may also feel a stretch along the outside of your body. Sit or stand holding the wand horizontally in front of you with the palm of your involved arm up and the other palm facing down. Without moving your trunk, move the wand across your body by raising your involved arm as high as possible. The wand will now be almost vertical. You will feel the stretch in your axilla and along the side of your trunk. Do not bend your trunk. Hold this stretch for fifteen seconds. Perform this in front of a mirror so you can watch to make sure you are not bending your trunk instead of raising your arm.

4. **Pectoral corner stretch.** This stretches the incision and skin across the chest wall as well as the pectoralis muscle. Tightness of the anterior chest or pectoralis muscle can affect your posture, pulling your shoulder forward and giving you a round-shouldered appearance. It can also make reaching out to the side or behind more difficult. When you do this correctly, you feel a stretch along the front of your chest and shoulder. Stand facing a corner. Place one hand and forearm on each wall with your elbows at shoulder level. Slowly lean your chest into the corner. You will feel a stretch across your chest wall. Hold this for fifteen seconds and return to the starting position. Keep your forearms flat against the wall throughout the movement.

    You can also do this starting with your elbows slightly above shoulder level. Slowly lean your chest into the corner. You will feel a stretch across your chest wall, but in a slightly different place from the last exercise. Hold the stretch for fifteen seconds, then return to the starting position.

5. **Rocking for shoulder flexion.** Using your body weight as a force can help make stretching easier. This exercise stretches your

axilla and the back of your arm. Get down on your hands and knees, with your hands positioned slightly in front of your shoulders. Place most of your weight on your legs and unaffected arm. (Don't do this exercise if placing weight on your affected shoulder causes pain.) Slowly rock back to your heels until you begin to feel a stretch in your shoulders. Hold this position for twenty to thirty seconds, then return to starting position. As the stretch becomes easier, start with your arms farther out in front of your body to increase the stretch.

Gentle Strengthening Exercises

Movement and skeletal muscle contraction provide a compression force on the veins and lymphatic vessels. This helps to facilitate and accelerate lymph flow in the arm. These exercises require handheld weights, but do not use weights that exceed three pounds each. Heavy weights are not necessary to create a compressive force and may even be harmful. Do not overdo. More is not always better. Ten to twenty repetitions a day will maintain muscle tone and facilitate lymph flow. It is normal for your muscles to be sore at the beginning of a strengthening program. Pace yourself. Do different exercises each day in order to give each area a rest after a workout. If your lymphedema begins to worsen, do fewer repetitions of the strengthening exercises. Resume them slowly as your arm improves. If increased swelling persists, consult your doctor or physical therapist. If you have a compression sleeve, it may be helpful to wear it while performing these exercises.

1. **Bilateral shoulder flexion.** This exercise contracts a part of your deltoid (shoulder) muscle and other muscles that raise your arm overhead. The deltoid lymph pathway is an alternative route for lymph flow, and contracting your deltoid muscle helps facilitate lymph movement along this pathway. Raising your arms overhead opens up your axilla, helping to clear the pathway for lymph to flow. Stand, preferably in front of a

mirror, with your arms down by your sides holding weights. With your elbows straight, raise both arms up in front of you and over your head evenly. Go only as high as your involved shoulder will go. Lower both arms slowly.

2. **Bilateral shoulder abduction.** This exercise contracts part of the deltoid muscle, helping to move lymph along the alternative pathway. Stand with your arms by your sides holding weights with your palms facing forward. Simultaneously raise both arms out to the side until your arms are parallel to the floor. Hold for a few seconds, then slowly lower your arms.

3. **Elbow bending (flexion).** This works the biceps muscle (at the front of the upper arm), which helps bend the elbow. Performing exercises with the muscles of the hand and elbow can help move lymph trapped in the forearm. Sit in a straight-backed chair or stand. Hold a weight in your involved hand, keeping your arm by your side. Bend your elbow, bringing your hand toward your shoulder. Keep your upper arm still, making sure the motion comes from your elbow only. Slowly return to starting position.

4. **Elbow straightening (elbow extension).** This uses your triceps muscle (at the back of the upper arm) to straighten the elbow. It also helps promote the flow of lymph trapped in the forearm. Lie on your back and hold a weight in your involved hand. Bend your arm so that your elbow points up toward the ceiling and your hand is near your ear. Hold your upper arm still with your opposite hand. Slowly straighten your elbow until it is fully extended. Slowly bend your elbow to return to the start position.

What Else Can Aggravate Lymphedema?

If you are susceptible to lymphedema, the weather and your diet can affect it, too. Close, humid air causes fluid to stay in your body, while clear, high-pressure air has the opposite effect. So weather can make you feel better or worse. Fluctuations in air pressure as well as prolonged air travel can affect you. If you are planning to be in a plane, wear your lymphedema sleeve.

Alcohol and salt keep fluid in your body, so avoid these when your arm is swollen. Also avoid high-protein drinks, red meat, and foods with monosodium glutamate. And don't smoke. This causes your blood vessels to constrict and impede your lymphatic system.

Where Can I Get a Support Sleeve?

Your physician or physical therapist may keep a selection of support sleeves or compression sleeves in several sizes in the office for patients to try on. If not, they will be able to refer you to a pharmacy or medical supplier who carries lymphedema sleeves. Proper fit is important. If the sleeve is too small, it will cut off circulation and make your arm worse. If it's too big, it won't do any good. Start with your doctor and get a prescription for size. Custom-made sleeves can be ordered, but they are rarely necessary.

The sleeve looks like a support stocking. Wear it for a day or two until the swelling goes down. You may need more than one sleeve, because as your swelling diminishes, you should then wear a smaller sleeve. Support sleeves cost between $32 and $100 and are usually covered by medical insurance.

What to Do If You Injure Your Arm

If you get minor cuts or bruises, do what you would normally do. Clean out the area with soap and water and apply an antiseptic or antibiotic ointment. Cover the area with a dressing or bandage until it is healed. To avoid worrying about infection, carry a small tube of antiseptic ointment and a few bandages in your bag or makeup kit. This way, you can treat any cut or scrape immediately and forget about it. Watch for signs of infection — redness or swelling of the wound itself or swelling of your arm. More serious injuries, such as an insect bite or a scratch from a pet, need medical attention right away. You may need systemic antibiotics to prevent infection. Infection of the soft tissue is called cellulitis. This in turn leads to lymphedema (although lymphedema can happen for no apparent reason).

To reduce the chance of infection, avoid getting injections in or having blood drawn from the involved arm or hand. Wear gloves while doing any work that exposes you to cuts and scratches, such as gardening. Use an electric razor to avoid puncturing the skin under your arm, and don't cut your cuticles. Keep your arm covered when you are at risk of being stung by an insect or scratched by a pet.

If you fall or sprain your arm, get medical attention if you are in pain. Otherwise, pack the injury with ice to prevent swelling and then watch carefully. It may be a good idea to get an X ray to be sure there is no hairline fracture. Ignoring a serious injury could cause problems later. Remember, any injury can upset the vascular and lymphatic systems in your arm.

What to Do If You Get Lymphedema

Women have been advised to elevate their arm and squeeze a ball, but according to a recent Scandinavian study, this is not very effective. If the swelling is caused by an obvious infection from a deep cut or a bite, then your doctor will probably prescribe antibiotics.

Your doctor should always be informed if you develop lymphedema. But you can manage on your own, once you get used to the way your arm reacts. If you have no obvious trauma, such as an insect bite, and your arm begins to swell, get it moving. Do the range-of-motion exercises. Put on your support sleeve and wear it during your waking hours, even while you exercise. The manual lymph drainage (MLD) system of massage redirects the lymphatics in your skin. Light pressure is applied with a circular motion that gently pushes fluid up

your arm and into your upper body. A licensed physical therapist should show you this, because it is not an ordinary massage.

Where Can I Get Manual Lymph Drainage Massage?

Physical therapy with manual lymph drainage, prescribed by
your doctor and performed by a licensed physical therapist,
focuses on gently massaging, with a pumping motion. This
stimulates the weakened lymphatic system by pushing the
stagnant fluid through the lymph vessels and helping to develop collateral channels through which the lymph can begin
to flow. A physical therapist can also help you learn how to
massage your own arm to help reduce swelling. Ask your
doctor, or the breast management team at your hospital, to
find out if there is a therapist trained in this technique. Medical insurance covers the cost of treatments with a licensed
therapist but not with a masseuse.

What If These Methods Don't Help?

If lymphedema persists despite exercise, the support sleeve, or
MLD, a sequential pneumatic pump can be used at your doctor's office or hospital. Air fills the sleeve that is fitted over
your arm and presses it against your arm, similar to the way a
blood pressure cuff works. The sleeve is inflated in sequentially
overlapping air compartments when the pump is turned on.
Pressure is heaviest at your fingers and eases off as it gets closer
to your shoulder.

These pumps can be purchased for home use, but they cost
thousands of dollars and are rarely necessary. If you need the
pump, rent or borrow one from a medical supply store or
hospital. Avoid the pump if you have heart disease. Your heart
may be stressed by the fluid returning into the system or any
blood clots that could be dislodged by the process and cause
more serious problems.

To Learn More About Lymphedema

Your doctor or your hospital physical therapy department can give you more information about lymphedema. Or you can contact the National Lymphedema Network, a nonprofit center established to provide information and guidance to patients and healthcare professionals. They have a counseling hotline program, referral service to medical and therapeutic treatment centers in your area, information on locating or establishing local support groups, and a periodic newsletter. They may also be able to refer you to low-cost treatment.

* **Breast Cancer Physical Therapy Center**   **215-772-0160**
1905 Spruce Street
Philadelphia, PA 19103
Call or write for the booklet *Recovery in Motion*, an exercise program to assist in the management of lymphedema. These exercises help you develop flexibility and strength. Linda Miller, founder of the center, specializes in breast rehabilitation and has helped set up nine breast rehabilitation centers in the United States.

* **National Lymphedema Network Hotline**   **800-541-3259**
2211 Post Street, Suite 404
San Francisco, CA 94115

✔ Questions to Ask About Lymphedema

These questions are meant to help you interview physicians and other healthcare professionals so that you can feel secure about your treatment decisions. Some of these questions have no clear-cut answers, some do. But ask anyway!

How do I know when my arm is swollen enough to suspect lymphedema?

Usually, if the circumference of your arm is more than half an inch larger than your other arm, or than your baseline measurement. You will notice your sleeves getting tight.

Which doctor should I call if I suspect I have lymphedema?

Your surgeon is the one most familiar with any condition related to surgery. In some cases, when the radiation or medical oncologist is treating you, he or she may be more involved. If you develop lymphedema after your treatment and follow-up care have ended, your family doctor may be the first one you call.

How much exercise is necessary to avoid lymphedema?

You may want to do range-of-motion exercises with your arm for the rest of your life to keep it in shape. If you are active and involved in regular exercise, that may be all you need. If your arm swells at all, you may want to focus on the special exercises for lymphedema.

My involved arm is also my dominant arm, so isn't it normally bigger than the other one?

Your dominant arm may normally be slightly larger than the other because it is more muscular from use. But the difference is usually slight. Again, the half-inch difference is a good gauge. Lymphedema involves swelling of skin and superficial tissue and not the muscle. You should be able to tell the difference by pressing your fingers into your arm. Your fingers can leave an impression in swollen tissue.

Will carrying heavy bags or a briefcase cause lymphedema?

This is an individual judgment, and some medical professionals think "hanging" weight is especially risky. If you are strong and fit, anything you normally do should be okay. In the past, some physicians have advised against hard resistance, such as pushing or carrying. If you are not strong, then carrying heavy weights won't feel good. Heavy lifting or pushing could also give you a hernia!

When should I use the support sleeve?

Whenever you feel your arm is beginning to swell. By using the sleeve right away, you discourage the collection of fluids in your arm.

Should I massage at the first sign of swelling?

Current thinking about lymphedema advises a combination of actions at the earliest sign of trouble. Wear your sleeve, do range-of-motion exercises, and use the manual lymph drainage massage, if you know how to do it. Massage by itself is not enough, and if you are not doing the MLD technique, then you are wasting your time.

~ 15

You *Will* Be Healthy — and Sexy — After Breast Cancer

We've noticed over the years how so many of our patients become stronger and happier after their breast cancer because they take better care of themselves. They pay more attention to diet and exercise and what's important in their lives. They reassess their priorities, maximize what they already have, and get rid of what's not working for them. Breast cancer is a frightening experience, and it can shake you into a more focused and dynamic lifestyle. Recovery is really about learning how to live — really live — no matter how many months or years are left.

Linda Creed wrote the hit song "The Greatest Love of All" after breast cancer. One of our patients, a teacher, had always wanted to write children's books. After breast cancer she started. Some women have suddenly gotten the courage, after breast cancer, to end bad marriages or relationships, or go out and find great ones!

A Primer on Nutrition and Weight Control

Disregard what we told you about diet in the chemotherapy chapter. There we recommended lots of calories — any calories — to cope with the cytotoxic drugs. Now that you are recovering, a well-balanced diet, low in fat and high in fiber with plenty of fresh fruits and vegetables, will keep you fit.

The National Cancer Institute believes a third of all cancers are related to diet, and the American Cancer Society found that the fatter you are, the greater your risk for cancer of the breast, uterus, gallbladder, kidney, stomach, and colon. Being obese — 40 percent above your ideal weight — puts you at the highest risk. Obese women have a lower survival with breast cancer than thinner women. Carrying too much body fat triggers a rise in estrogen, which is known to fuel the growth of some tumors.

The irony, of course, is that some breast cancer therapy can cause weight gain. Tamoxifen, for example, is a powerful appetite stimulant and makes you feel hungry — really hungry. Most people taking tamoxifen will gain 10 to 15 pounds. Sometimes cytotoxic chemotherapy is an indirect cause of weight gain. By constantly snacking to fight off low-grade nausea for months, you gain weight. Fluid retention is another by-product of chemotherapy.

To maintain your proper weight, eat well, count calories, and exercise. There is no magic way to lose weight. Calculate your ideal weight by adding 5 pounds to 100 for every inch you are over five feet tall. If you are five feet seven, you should weigh 135 pounds, give or take a few pounds for different bone and body structure. So if you weigh 155 and should weigh 135, you are 11 percent overweight. If you are more than 25 percent overweight, it's unhealthy.

What Is the Truth About Fat and Breast Cancer?

The controversy about whether or not high-fat diets cause breast cancer continues. Some researchers say no, others insist dietary fat is a factor. We may not know for sure just how — whether fat starts cancer or speeds the growth of an already existing cancer — but we cannot abandon the link between dietary fat and breast cancer. In countries where fat consumption is low, there is less breast cancer.

A 1993 Swedish study reported in the *Journal of the National Cancer Institute* implies that reducing fat intake may act like adjuvant therapy. Two hundred twenty women with positive estrogen receptors, who had surgery for breast cancer, and who consumed diets with saturated fats accounting for more than 17.5 percent of daily calories, ran a 20 percent higher risk of breast cancer recurring. Each 1 percent increase in fat calories was associated with an approximately 8 percent increase in disease recurrence. The implications of this study are that dietary fat may in fact enhance the growth of some types of breast cancer.

The most well known and controversial study of the relationship between fat and breast cancer is the Nurses Health Study conducted at the Harvard School of Public Health. The average American diet of 40 percent fat was compared with a 30 percent fat diet, and the findings indicated that the diet made no difference in occurrence of breast cancer. However, 30 percent of calories from fat is not a low-fat diet. Low-fat is 20 percent or less.

The Women's Health Initiative study sponsored by the National Institutes of Health is now following 70,000 postmenopausal women to find out if a diet high in vegetables and grains, with only 20 percent of calories from fat, can reduce the risk of breast cancer. Results are not yet in, but we believe this to be the healthiest way to eat.

Whatever is true about fat and breast cancer, too much fat is not good for your heart and blood vessels, your cholesterol level, or your colon. While animal fat is considered more harmful than vegetable oils, too much of any fat is bad.

Saturated fat becomes solid at room temperature because it is full of hydrogen. Most saturated fat is animal fat, except for palm and coconut oils, which are also saturated fats. Margarine is a vegetable oil made solid (and saturated) by adding hydrogen, so too much of it is just as harmful as too much butter. A tablespoon of any fat is about 100 calories.

The worst thing about fat in the diet — any fat — is that it is addictive. (So is salt.) It will take time to withdraw — probably about three months. Don't expect miracles of yourself. When you try to curb your hunger with an apple rather than a bowl of ice cream, your fat cells will be screaming for satisfaction. If your recommended daily intake is 2,000 calories, then you can have only 400 fat calories a day — or 44.4 grams of fat — on a 20 percent fat diet. Get an inexpensive pocket guide that lists calories and fat grams for a variety of foods. Many are available in bookstores or free from health agencies such as the American Cancer Society and the American Heart Association. There are new cookbooks appearing all the time with low-fat, high-fiber menus.

How Is Fiber Related to Breast Cancer?

Without enough fiber in your diet, food takes two to three times longer to pass through your body. This means harmful bacteria are hanging around in your digestive tract and leaning on your intestine walls long enough to cause trouble. We know fiber reduces the risk of colon cancer. But some investigators now believe that fiber in the diet also encourages the creation of the less dangerously reactive form of estrogen and may impede breast cancer.

High-fiber foods include cereals, grains, beans, fruit, and vegetables. Most raw fruits and vegetables have more useful fiber than those that have been peeled, blended, cooked, or processed. Whole-wheat bread has more fiber than white bread; an orange, more than its juice. The downside is that fiber, if you are not used to it, can cause gas and bloating. This is a normal reaction, so increase fiber gradually in your diet. Eat well-balanced meals and this will subside in a few weeks.

More Good Reasons to Eat Vegetables

Vegetables and fruit are not only good sources of fiber, they contain other elements that play a role in disease prevention. People who eat lots of plant food seem less prone to get cancer than meat eaters. Chemists analyzing vegetables have discovered many properties that have implications for cancer research. Some of these ingredients retard the cell breakdowns that result in cancer. Scientists have agreed that carotene and antioxidants in vegetables are important in protecting your body against an assortment of ills — including cancer.

Cruciferous vegetables. You can't cure breast cancer by eating pounds of broccoli every day, but a healthy diet that includes sufficient amounts of cruciferous vegetables like broccoli, brussels sprouts, bok choy, cabbage, cauliflower, collards, and turnips, could very well impede the growth of cancer. There may be an element in cruciferous vegetables that induces estrogen to remain in its inert state rather than the active state that is implicated in tumors. This is the same inert form found in high levels in female athletes. The Strang-Cornell Cancer Research Laboratory in New York is studying how plant chemicals influence estrogen metabolism and thus how diet might inhibit breast cancer.

We know that estradiol, the precursor to estrogen, can turn into an active (16-hydroxylated) or inert (2-hydroxylated) form. Women with a high risk of breast cancer show elevated levels of the 16 type in their blood. Breast tumor tissue contains more of the 16-hydroxylated form than does the surrounding noncancerous breast tissue. One chemical in particular, indole-3-carbinol, induces estradiol to follow the harmless metabolic route toward 2-hydroxylation.

A study of sixty women taking daily capsules of 400 milligrams of indole carbinol, the equivalent of half a head of cabbage, shows that within weeks their levels of the harmless 2-hydroxylated estrogen had risen to concentrations seen in marathon runners. Lower doses of the compound are being tested on larger groups of women, but it will be years before we learn exactly how the difference in estrogen metabolism affects breast cancer rates.

Another vegetable element, genisten, found in soybeans (a good reason to eat lots of tofu) and some cruciferous vegetables, blocks angiogenesis — the growth of new blood vessels. If this could be used in treatment, it could prevent cancer cells from developing new capillaries that supply blood to tumors. Sulforaphane, which is found in broccoli, appears to be an anticancer agent. This and other so-called isothiocyanates found in cruciferous vegetables seem to stimulate production of protective enzymes in the body.

Carotene and vitamin A. There appears to be universal agreement on the importance of vitamin A and carotene. Women who ate less than one serving a day of food high in vitamin A had a 20 percent higher risk of breast cancer. Eating one or two servings a day was enough to cancel the higher risk. However, the risk was not reduced by taking large amounts of vitamin A supplements, only by the nutrient coming from food. These findings came from the same nurses study used for the high-fat comparisons, in which 89,000 women were followed for eight years. Carotene is a precursor of vitamin A, that is, it becomes vitamin A when metabolized in your body. The best sources are orange, green, and yellow vegetables: carrots, sweet potatoes, cantaloupes, yellow squash, and spinach. The deeper the color — usually orange and dark green — the more carotenoids a vegetable has. Pumpkin has more than yellow summer squash. Kale and spinach have more than lettuce.

Antioxidants. While we are breathing and burning up energy, our cells continuously generate hazardous waste that can set the stage for cancer. This waste is made of molecules known as free radicals. Most free radicals are mopped up by our body's own police force — antioxidant enzymes. However, without proper diet, our antioxidant levels can be low. Vitamins A, C, and E and beta carotene are all antioxidants. Good sources are melons and citrus fruits, yellow and green vegetables, tomatoes, green leafy vegetables, potatoes, wheat germ, oatmeal, peanuts, and brown rice. Broccoli and garlic are especially rich in antioxidants. In fact, the National Cancer Institute puts garlic high on its list of natural antioxidants. Eaten raw, garlic also stimulates immunological functions, lowers blood cholesterol, thins blood, and helps prevent embolisms.

The scientific community has only just begun to study our diets, and there are many things we don't know. There could be elements in vegetables that *give* us cancer, too, but the positive benefits appear to far outweigh any potential hazards. And keep in mind that vegetables can have more or less of these good elements depending on how they were grown, stored, and cooked.

Alcohol and Breast Cancer

Alcohol has been implicated in breast cancer, so moderation is wise. Because we have more body fat, women don't metabolize alcohol as well as men. A study by the National Cancer Institute showed that premenopausal women taking two drinks a day had a shift in estrogen hormones that could be the mechanism behind the rise in breast cancer associated with alcohol. So moderate alcohol may be good for your heart, but not good for breast cancer. In the Harvard nurses study, women who typically consumed three to nine drinks a week were 30 percent more likely than nondrinkers to develop breast cancer. Other studies go so far as to say one drink a day increases the risk by 10 percent and two drinks by 25 percent. Ironically, a glass of red wine with dinner every day could actually make you feel better. It contains an antioxidant substance that prevents cholesterol from clogging the arteries. So if you do have a drink, try that.

Becoming Addicted to Exercise

Exercise lowers estrogen production, which is why athletes often stop menstruating, and it is believed to reduce the risk of breast cancer. It also strengthens your heart and lungs, helps prevent osteoporosis, and lifts your spirits. Lean body weight is associated with improved breast cancer prognosis. Exercise directed toward range of motion as well as muscle strength and cardiovascular fitness should become part of your daily routine.

A woman who had breast cancer in the 1970s and endured nearly two years of chemotherapy recalls how she got turned on to exercise: "I knew I had to do something, but running was boring. Aerobics classes and swimming pools were not available, I couldn't afford to play tennis. I went around asking my friends, 'What should I do?' Finally, one of them asked me, 'What did you like as a kid?' I liked riding my bike. There it was! I began with short rides around the neighborhood and eventually went on bike hikes with other cyclists." This woman is now an international cyclist who has biked her way around the world.

Even if you walk every day for half an hour, this will help you stay fit. Everything helps. Walking is one of the best cardiovascular exercises. Walk as quickly as you can, with your arms swinging. Start slowly and let it become part of your life. When your body gets used to exercising it will crave it, and soon a good habit will develop. You need at least twenty minutes of vigorous exercise three times a week. If you exercise for longer than twenty minutes at a time, you'll start to burn off calories.

ENCORE. The national YWCA sponsors ENCORE, a program for postoperative breast cancer patients, which includes exercise to music, water exercises, and a discussion period. You can join the third week after surgery with your doctor's permission. For information, check the YWCA in your area. ENCORE stands for Encouragement, Normalcy, Counseling, Opportunity, Reaching Out, Energies Revived.

Working out. If you are disciplined enough, try an aerobic exercise video and work out at home. Otherwise, consider joining a class. If you have access to a health club or YWCA, there's a good beginning. Health clubs are no longer the domain of bodybuilders. People of all ages and conditions participate in fitness programs these days. Treadmills, stationary bicycles, stairclimbers, rowing machines, are all metered to tell you how much work you are doing. The best machines for cardiovascular fitness put your large muscles in motion.

Active sports. If you are an athlete, there is no reason why you cannot continue to be one, once your doctors give you the all clear after treatment. It may take a period of time to regain your strength. But be persistent. Look to the long term and your way of life. We know of a runner over forty who had a mastectomy and went back to competing for the Olympic tryouts. Every sport includes breast cancer survivors.

Physical therapy. There are physical therapists at some cancer centers and independents who specialize in reconditioning breast cancer patients. You may have a greater need than some for physical therapy after surgery and radiation because you have more tightness, especially after recurrence and radiation. Whoever gives you physical therapy should have knowledge of and experience with breast cancer patients and know how to work out a threefold program: first, to restore range of motion, then to bring your involved muscles up to 100 percent fitness, and, finally, to get the rest of your body in shape.

When You Should *Stop* Exercising

There are times during treatment when exercise could be harmful. You should not exercise within twenty-four hours of receiving intravenous chemotherapy, or if you have been nauseated or have vomited in the past twenty-four to thirty-six hours. You may be dehydrated and therefore too weak to tolerate exercise. Any of the following symptoms would also be a signal to stop exercising:

- unusual fatigue or muscle weakness
- irregular pulse
- pain or cramps in your legs
- chest pain
- nausea during exercise
- feeling disoriented, confused, faint, or dizzy
- blurred vision
- pale complexion (pallor cyanosis)
- sudden shortness of breath
- decreasing heart rate and blood pressure despite the increased workload

Intimate Relationships and Breast Cancer

If you had a good sex life before breast cancer, there's no reason you can't have one now. Even if you didn't have one before, there's always hope for the future. If you have an affectionate partner who has been supportive (not to be confused with guilt-ridden) throughout your treatment, you probably will have no problems.

However, you may feel self-conscious about your changed body, or apprehensive about injuring yourself. Your partner may also be afraid of hurting you. Talk to each other. Openly communicating your feelings to each other is the best way.

If you are tender or sore or feel any physical discomfort, try new methods. Experiment. But most important is the affection and caring. Don't feel pressured to perform. You need love and affection right now. So if it feels good, do it. If it hurts, stop and try some other way.

There are many men who are simply unable or unwilling to cope with breast cancer. They usually leave the scene. In that case, well, good riddance. If a man is willing to learn how to cope, there are many resources available. He can start with individual counseling or a support group for men or families of breast cancer survivors. The husband of actress Ann Jillian coauthored a book to help men understand what their women are going through. Y-ME recently published a booklet, *When the Woman You Love Has Breast Cancer*, which can be obtained from the national office. (See Appendix 4.)

For every man who cannot cope, there is another who can. Two patients who were diagnosed just before they were to be married had husbands-to-be who were very supportive, and these couples are still together. Another patient was dating when she had her first mastectomy, married, then had a second mastectomy, and is now coping with infertility. She and her husband are planning to adopt a child. A patient with bilateral mastectomy with implant reconstruction is dating a younger man — and quite happy about it!

When Is It Safe to Get Pregnant?

What about getting pregnant after you've had breast cancer? In general, women are advised to wait two to five years, if possible, since these years represent the time when the risk for recurrence (local and systemic) is highest. Pregnancy upsets your hormones, and it's hard to predict what will happen. If you are over thirty and have chemotherapy, you also face the possibility of early menopause.

One patient we know who completed treatment when she was thirty-five waited five years and at forty gave birth to a beautiful baby. Another, a thirty-eight-year-old, is trying now for a baby, a year and a half after completing treatment. Yet another woman had a small local recurrence after radiation therapy, had it treated, then a year later had a baby. She and her baby are fine. Although many doctors would not recommend nursing because the breast becomes engorged and difficult to examine, some women have done it. One new mother breast-fed her baby for four months with some milk production in the radiated breast.

In Closing

You can have children after breast cancer. You can have anything you want after breast cancer. We are very proud of the way our patients have come through their struggles with this disease, how they have recovered with renewed strength and determination to lead healthier, happier, and more fulfilling lives.

We hope this book helps you learn what you need to know to get the best treatment you can find. There is a great deal of information available now about breast cancer that was not available in the past. Take advantage of all the resources at your disposal. Use this book and share it with others who may need it. Communicate with the women in your support group and with your families and friends. And above all, communicate with your doctors. Ask them questions. Ask for better explanations if you are not sure you understand. It makes us feel better when you feel better. After all, we chose to treat breast cancer because we wanted to make a difference.

Every day we learn more about treating breast cancer, and one day we will find a way to prevent it. We hope that day will be in our lifetime.

∼ Appendix 1

Sources of Financial Aid for Breast Cancer Treatment

Where to Get Free or Low-Cost Mammograms

Many communities have hospitals or private foundations that periodically provide free or low-cost mammograms and early detection opportunities. The Linda Creed Breast Cancer Foundation in Philadelphia (215-955-4354) provides free mammograms once a month at various healthcare sites. Some corporations sponsor free mammograms and BSE classes for employees as well as underserved women in their communities. These include Avon, Liz Claiborne, DuPont, Adolph Coors, and Merck & Company. Check with your employer's health office, the social service department of your hospital, or call the local office of the American Cancer Society (ACS) to find out what's available in your area. October is National Breast Cancer Awareness month and there may be more free screenings available then.

Financial Aid for Chemotherapy

Drug companies often provide chemotherapy drugs at low or no cost to people who cannot afford to pay for them. Your chemotherapist or your local ACS chapter may know about this. Your chemotherapist can also write for the Directory of Prescription Drug Indigent Programs, which can help locate drugs at low or no cost. This is published by the Pharmaceutical Manufacturers Association in Washington, D.C.

Funding Experimental Treatment

The Noreen T. Holland Breast Cancer Foundation in New York sometimes provides money for experimental treatment. The foundation's primary focus is funding research to find ways to prevent breast cancer. Call them at 914-381-3050 in Mamaroneck, or write P.O. Box One, Oyster Bay, NY 11771.

Overcoming Medical Insurance Limitations

Medical insurance coverage varies, and even if you are fully covered, you may still have to pay a percentage of the charges yourself. There may also be a limit to your coverage, and after that limit has been reached, you are responsible for the rest of the payment. Most treatment centers and hospitals have three sets of figures for each patient procedure: What they charge the patient; what the treatment costs them to give you; and what they will receive from medical insurance companies. For this reason, there is some flexibility, and you can probably negotiate a fair price in advance if you know you are going to have to come up with an enormous amount of money. So the advice here is to find out what all the charges are, how much your insurance will cover, and what remains for you to pay.

Transportation To and From Treatments

Again, ask the local ACS chapter or your treatment team about transportation resources. They can also tell you about a national Corporate Angels program that provides long-distance air transportation to a treatment facility.

~ Appendix 2

Your Right to See Your Medical Records

Federal law guarantees your right to your medical records. It also protects your right of privacy, so that others cannot have your medical records without your knowledge and approval. Most hospitals have a medical records department; these departments sometimes move slowly because a great deal of paper is handled there. If you want a copy of any or all of your medical records, you have to put the request in writing and complete a form supplied by the hospital. This legally protects both you and the hospital. You should be able to get copies of your records within a few days, however, and sooner if it is urgent. You are entitled to hospital records, doctor records, diagnostic records, X-ray films, pathology slides, all of it.

Your records are your files and you will want to have them — or at least know what's in them — if you visit other doctors or hospitals. You don't need the full set of records. The most useful are your pathology, mammography, and operative reports. You may want them with you so that years later you will have easy access to them if you need them. You may want your family or other significant people to be able to get your medical information in an emergency.

∼ Appendix 3

Will You Be Able to Keep or Change Jobs (and Get Health Insurance)?

In 1993, the Equal Employment Opportunity Commission (EEOC) declared that employers cannot refuse to hire people with disabilities and that these people must have equal access to health insurance. The agency also said it would enforce the 1990 Americans with Disabilities Act to curb discrimination by employers and insurers.

Enforcement is necessary because this kind of discrimination is often disguised. People are laid off if employers think they will need more benefits or be out sick often. One woman who had a mastectomy shortly before she turned sixty-five was forced to retire at sixty-five even though she wanted to continue working. The end of work also meant the end of benefits for her, yet when she questioned the employer (a hospital, no less!), she was told that a mandatory retirement ruling had been established. She was deprived of her benefits as well as a job she had planned to enjoy for several more years.

The first thing to do in a case like this is talk with the affirmative action officer at work and let him or her know that you believe you were unjustly laid off. The company cannot retaliate by firing you. Look for comparisons. Was another employee allowed to return after a heart attack? If you are not reinstated, file a complaint with your state human rights commission within 180 days and the EEOC within 300 days. Find a plaintiff's attorney to help you file this. Very often, an attorney will take on this kind of case without a fee and then get a percentage of the settlement later.

The new law relates to present and future jobs. If you are turned down for a new job for reasons you believe are false, you should protest. Don't discuss your health at a job interview. A prospective employer cannot ask about your health until you are given the job. When you fill out forms for medical insurance, do not accept the exclusion clause for breast disorders. Some insurance companies are already beginning to eliminate the "preexisting conditions" clause in coverage. Look for a policy that allows you to choose your physicians and place of treatment. Do not compromise your treatment options.

The American Cancer Society has a booklet explaining the Americans with Disabilities Act and your legal rights pertaining to jobs and health insurance. Call your local chapter for a copy.

∽ Appendix 4

Hotlines for Information About Breast Cancer

There is a growing network of information available about breast cancer. People who answer telephone hotlines are trained to provide information on breast cancer. Most of these agencies can provide information in Spanish as well as English. If you call with a question or need a referral, they can help you. If they can't, they will know who can.

American Cancer Society   **800-ACS-2345 for your local chapter**
This is the largest voluntary health agency in the world, with 3,400 chapters in the United States. ACS sponsors research, education, and patient service programs, including transportation to and from treatment, equipment loans, volunteer visitor programs such as Reach to Recovery, and support groups. Your local chapter is usually a good place to find out what resources are available in your community. Two affiliated programs:

- **Look Good, Feel Better**   **800-395-LOOK, or local ACS**
Hotline operated weekdays between 9 A.M. and 5 P.M. eastern standard time. Referrals to free workshops in fifty states that provide practical advice from hair and makeup professionals. Brochures and information in English and Spanish. Founded in 1989 and developed by the

Cosmetic, Toiletry, and Fragrance Association Foundation, in cooperation with the American Cancer Society and the National Cosmetology Association.

- **Reach to Recovery.** Volunteer breast cancer survivors are trained by ACS to meet and talk with breast cancer patients. The volunteer who visits you is often someone who had the same kind of treatment. She can show you how to wear a breast prosthesis, or talk with you about reconstruction. Reach to Recovery also offers separate support groups for lumpectomy and mastectomy patients.

American College of Surgeons Committee on Cancer
55 East Erie Street
Chicago, IL 60611

Write for a booklet listing approved cancer programs. Revised quarterly.

American Society of Plastic and Reconstructive
Surgeons   800-635-0635
444 East Algonquin Road
Arlington Heights, IL 60005

A twenty-four-hour referral line. Leave a message asking for board-certified plastic and reconstructive surgeons in your area. They will send you five names and an educational brochure within seven days. Also leave the name of a particular physician to find out if he or she is board certified and a member of the society. For other questions, call weekdays between 8:30 A.M. and 4:30 P.M. central time.

The BMT Newsletter   708-831-1913
1985 Spruce Avenue
Highland Park, IL 60035

A bimonthly publication with information from those who have had bone marrow transplant.

Breast Cancer Physical Therapy Center   215-772-0160
1905 Spruce Street
Philadelphia, PA 19103

For a booklet on exercises to help manage lymphedema. Cost is $8.95, which includes shipping.

Breast Implant Information Line   800-532-4440

>   Established by the Food and Drug Administration in 1992 to answer
>   questions about the safety of breast implants. They will send a
>   current information package, instructions on how to enroll in a
>   clinical study, and a list of questions to ask your surgeon before you
>   have implant reconstruction.

The Chemotherapy Foundation   212-213-9292
183 Madison Avenue
New York, NY 10016

>   Ask for a list of certified medical oncologists in your area and for
>   their free booklet on chemotherapy and breast cancer.

ENCORE   **Call your local YWCA**

>   Sponsored by the national YWCA, this program for postoperative
>   breast cancer patients includes exercise to music, water exercises,
>   and a discussion period. You can join on the third week after surgery
>   with your doctor's permission. For information, check the YWCA in
>   your area. ENCORE stands for Encouragement, Normalcy, Counsel-
>   ing, Opportunity, Reaching Out, Energies Revived.

Linda Creed Breast Cancer Foundation   215-955-4354

>   Based in Philadelphia, home of songwriter Linda Creed, who died
>   of breast cancer at age thirty-eight. Provides free mammograms for
>   disadvantaged women once a month. Also has education programs
>   and support groups for breast cancer patients, and is involved in
>   political advocacy and fund-raising.

NABCO Hotline   212-719-0154
National Alliance of Breast Cancer Organizations
1180 Avenue of the Americas
New York, NY 10036

>   NABCO is an encyclopedia of breast cancer resources for patients
>   and healthcare professionals. Its annual *Breast Cancer Resource List*
>   is $3 and includes comprehensive listings of everything available,
>   including phone numbers for the more than three hundred support
>   groups in the nation. NABCO publishes fact sheets on current and
>   new treatment and research, and a periodic newsletter for members.
>   Materials are available in Spanish.

National Bone Marrow Transplant Link   800-LINK-BMT
29209 Northwestern Highway, No. 624
Southfield, MI 48034

An information clearinghouse and link with other patients and families of patients.

National Lymphedema Network Hotline   800-541-3259
2211 Post Street, Suite 404
San Francisco, CA 94115

For referrals for medical treatment, physical therapy, general information, and support in your area. They will send you an information packet.

NCI Cancer Information Service Hotline   800-4-CANCER

The National Cancer Institute (NCI) is the primary federal agency for cancer research and information on everything from clinical trials to new drugs. The hotline is operated by a network of authorized comprehensive cancer centers. When you dial, you'll be connected with the one nearest you. They keep a file of available resources and physicians working with many types of cancer and can refer in all specialties.

Nolvadex (Tamoxifen) Information and Service   800-456-5678

This is an information service operated by the company that manufactures tamoxifen. They will answer questions and send you information.

Y-ME National Hotline   800-221-2141

Chicago-based Y-ME provides a national and regional hotlines, as well as referrals for medical care and information on finding or starting support groups. Phone calls are answered by breast cancer survivors weekdays between 9 A.M. and 5 P.M. central time. They maintain a wig and prosthesis bank for women who cannot afford them. There are eighteen chapters in the United States and Canada. The regional phone numbers are:

California, Sacramento area	**916-921-9747**
California, San Francisco Bay area	**408-261-1425**
Chicago and emergencies (24 hours)	**708-799-8228**

Connecticut (statewide)   800-933-4YME
Maryland, West Virginia,
    Virginia (703), Pennsylvania (717)   800-963-0101
Massachusetts   413-243-4822
South Dakota   605-339-HELP
Washington, D.C., and Virginia   703-461-9616

∼ Appendix 5

Some Helpful Reading

Cancer and Nutrition, by Charles B. Simone, M.D. (Garden City Park, N.Y.: Avery, 1992).

> Written by a doctor who believes nutrition makes a big difference.

Dr. Susan Love's Breast Book, by Susan M. Love, M.D., and Karen Lindsey (Reading, Mass.: Addison-Wesley, 1990).

> This is like an encyclopedia of the breast and will tell you all you want to know about how your breasts work and what can go wrong with them.

Earl Mindell's Vitamin Bible, by Earl Mindell (New York: Warner, 1994).

> All you need to know about the nutrients in your food and how they affect you.

Prescription for Nutritional Healing, by James Balch, M.D., and Phyllis Balch, C.N.C. (Garden City Park, N.Y.: Avery, 1990).

> Another look at nutrition and good health.

The Race Is Run One Step at a Time: Every Woman's Guide to Taking Charge of Breast Cancer, by Nancy Brinker and Catherine Harris (New York: Simon & Schuster, 1991).

A Woman's Decision: Breast Care, Treatment, and Reconstruction, by Karen Berger and John Bostwick, III (St. Louis: Quality Medical Publishing, 1993).

Comprehensive information about reconstruction and stories from women who have been through it.

Women Talk About Breast Surgery: From Diagnosis to Recovery, by Amy Gross and Dee Ito (New York: HarperCollins, 1991).

More stories from women.

Glossary

Adenopathy. Enlarged lymph nodes; may suggest presence of breast cancer. Also called lymphadenopathy.

Adjuvant therapy. Additional treatment given at the same time as or after the primary therapy.

Adriamycin. Brand name for doxorubicin, a cytotoxic drug used to treat breast cancer. The "A" in CAF (see entry). Can have some toxicity to heart, often associated with hair loss.

Alopecia. Hair loss.

Aneuploid. Term used to describe a cell population that contains other than the normal amount of DNA material.

Areola. The flattened area of dark skin around the nipple of the breast.

Atypical hyperplasia. Excessive growth of cells; a premalignant condition. May be ductal or lobular.

Autologous. From the same person, as in autologous bone marrow transplantation, autologous flap in breast reconstruction, autologous blood transfusion.

Axilla. The underarm.

Axillary dissection. Surgical removal of lymph nodes from under the arm.

Axillary tail. Extreme tip of the breast that extends into armpit area.

Benign. Not cancerous; nonmalignant.

Bilateral mastectomy. Surgical removal of both breasts.

Biofeedback. A method of self-monitoring and controlling some bodily systems. Used to reduce muscle tension, blood pressure, nausea, stress, pain.

Biopsy. Removal of tissue for histologic analysis, microscopic study, or pathologic evaluation. Can remove cells (needle aspiration, needle cytology), part of lesion (incisional biopsy), or all of lesion (excisional biopsy).

Boost. Term used in radiation treatment to indicate the dose of radiation delivered directly to the tumor site.

Breast conservation. Surgical removal of a tumor without removing the breast; lumpectomy.

BSE. Breast self-examination.

CA15-3. A blood test to find cancer recurrence or metastasis. More suggestive of bone metastasis.

CA125. A blood test mostly used to check for breast and ovarian cancer.

CAF. Combination of cytotoxic drugs used in chemotherapy — Cytoxan, Adriamycin, fluorouracil.

Calcifications. Deposits of calcium in the soft tissue of the breast. Seen on mammography, often in the absence of a palpable mass, but can indicate presence of malignancy, depending on clustering, pattern, shape, and number.

Capsular contracture. Scar tissue that forms around a breast implant.

Carcinoma. Cancer that begins in the lining or covering tissues of an organ (epithelium), such as breast ducts.

CAT scan. Computerized axial tomography. A cross-sectional X ray used in diagnosis and radiation treatment planning.

CEA. A blood test to look for metastasis.

Cellulitis. An infection of the soft tissue.

Chemotherapy. Systemic treatment with medications that reach every cell in the body. Can be cytotoxic (see entry) or hormonal.

Clavicle. Collarbone.

Clavicular. Around the collarbone, or clavicle.

Clinical trials. Controlled studies of cancer treatments on a fixed number of patients designed to answer certain questions.

CMF. Combination of cytotoxic drugs used in breast cancer chemotherapy — Cytoxan, methotrexate, fluorouracil.

Comedo carcinoma. A type of very early cancer starting in the breast ducts; thought to be more aggressive than other in situ cancer. Characterized by areas of necrosis.

CTX. Medical shorthand for "chemotherapy treatment."

Cyst. A fluid-filled mass or area; common in the breast and rarely associated with cancer.

Cytology. The study of cells under the microscope.

Cytotoxic. Toxic to cells. Refers to drugs used in chemotherapy to kill or slow down the reproduction of cancer cells.

Cytoxan. Brand name for cyclophosphamide, a cytotoxic drug used to treat breast cancer.

DCIS. See *ductal carcinoma in situ*.

Differentiation. The resemblance of cancer cells to normal cells. Well-differentiated tumor cells closely resemble normal cells and are, therefore, believed to be less aggressive.

Diffuse. Not concentrated or organized. Refers to cancer cells that are spread out, thinly scattered over a large area.

Diploid. Term to describe a cell population that contains the normal amount — 1.00 — of DNA material.

DNA. Deoxyribonucleic acid. Material in the cell nucleus (brain of the cell) that codes what that cell will become, its job.

Donor site. Part of the body from which skin (flap) is taken to graft onto the chest in breast reconstruction.

Doxorubicin. See *Adriamycin*.

Duct. A tubular structure in the breast through which milk passes to the nipple.

Ductal carcinoma in situ (DCIS). A breast cancer in the breast ducts that has not become invasive. Also called intraductal carcinoma.

Electrocautery. A surgical tool that utilizes electric current to cut and cauterize tissue. It is used to make incisions and stem blood flow.

Electron boost. Radiation focused on the tumor site from outside the breast with an electron beam, as opposed to an implant boost placed inside the breast tissue.

Epidermal growth factor receptors. Measurements of rate of tumor cell growth. Can be used along with hormone receptor analysis to gauge how patient will respond to hormone therapy.

ER/PR receptor analysis. A study to measure or detect the presence of estrogen and progesterone receptors in the tumor. The presence or absence of these receptors is important in determining if you need cytotoxic or hormone chemotherapy.

Estrogen. A female hormone usually and primarily produced by the ovaries.

Estrogen receptor. A protein on the tumor cell surface that binds with estrogen.

Excisional biopsy. Surgical biopsy that removes entire lesion.

External prosthesis. An artificial breast form worn outside the body, fitted inside clothing. Compare *implant*.

Extracapsular extension. A term used to indicate that cancer cells in a lymph node have extended through its outer coating into the surrounding fatty tissue.

Fibroadenoma. A benign growth found in the breast. The most common breast mass, particularly in younger women (from teens to thirties).

Film screen mammography. The most advanced form of mammography, uses films like X rays.

Flap. A piece of skin, muscle, and fat wholly or partially removed from one part of the body to use in breast reconstruction. See also *free flap, pedicle flap, TRAM flap*.

Flow cytometry. Analysis of tumor cells performed on biopsy specimens to determine the number of cells that are multiplying in order to try to determine how fast the tumor is growing.

Fluorouracil. Cytotoxic drug used to treat breast cancer. Also called 5-FU.

Free flap. A piece of tissue completely detached from another part of the body to use in breast reconstruction.

Frozen section. A small piece of a larger piece of tissue taken out during a biopsy that is flash frozen for instant analysis to determine whether cancer is present.

General anesthesia. Drugs that make you unconscious during surgery and usually require an endotracheal tube.

Genetic markers. Abnormalities found in the genes that indicate the potential to develop into, or the presence of, cancer.

Gluteus maximus. Muscle of the buttock, often used for breast reconstruction.

Grade. Classification of cancer that looks at the pattern of tumor cells and nuclei. Grade I describes the least aggressive forms of cancer, Grade III the most aggressive.

Histologic diagnosis. Study of tissue under the microscope, the most minute branch of anatomic study. The information in your pathology report.

Hormone receptor analysis. See *ER/PR receptor analysis*.

Hormone therapy. Treatment of cancer by blocking the ability of hormones to interact with cancer cells.

Hyperplasia. Excessive formation of cells.

Hyperthermia. The use of heat to kill or slow cancer cells. Most commonly used by radiation therapist particularly to treat chest wall recurrences or large, bulky tumors.

Implant. A prosthetic device placed under the skin. A silicone bag filled with saline (salt water) used for breast reconstruction.

Implant boost. A radioactive isotope implanted into the tumor site to give focused radiation. It is removed once the treatment is delivered.

Incisional biopsy. A surgical biopsy that removes a piece of tissue from the lesion.

Inflammatory breast cancer. An aggressive cancer that presents like an infection or inflammatory process and causes the breast to swell and redden. Accounts for about 1 percent of all breast cancers.

Infraclavicular. Term used to describe lymph nodes (or any condition) in the area below the collarbone.

Infusaport. See *port*.

Infusion. A method of delivering medications into the bloodstream gradually by using intravenous medications diluted with sugar water.

In situ cancer. A cancer that is "in place," noninvasive, and has not spread beyond that histologic structure. In situ ductal cancer, for example, is a cancer of ductal cells confined within the duct wall.

Intraductal carcinoma. Tumor within the breast ducts. DCIS.

Intramammary node. Lymph nodes found in the breasts.

Intravenous. Into or within the veins.

Invasive cancer. Cancer that can or has spread from its histologic original site. Invasive ductal cancer cells, for example, have broken through the duct walls and infiltrated the surrounding breast tissue.

Irradiation. Radiation therapy.

Latissimus dorsi. A large muscle of the back.

LCIS. See *lobular carcinoma in situ*.

Lesion. A tumor, mass, or other abnormality.

Lobe, lobule. Part of the breast involved in making milk.

Lobular carcinoma in situ (LCIS). Abnormal cell growth in the lobules; a premalignant condition often multicentric and bilateral. Also called lobular neoplasia.

Local anesthesia. A drug that numbs only an area of your body and allows you to remain awake.

Local treatment. In breast cancer cases, treatment aimed at the cells in the breast tumor and the area close to it.

Lumpectomy. Surgical removal of a tumor or lump from inside the breast without removing the breast. Usually more than excisional biopsy since it also includes a margin of normal tissue around the tumor. Also called breast conservation.

Lymph. Fluid that bathes body tissues and carries cells that help fight infection. The lymphatic system operates much like the circulatory system.

Lymphedema. Swelling of tissue (usually of the hand or arm in breast cancer cases) caused by extra fluid that may collect in tissues when lymph nodes are removed or blocked. Can also be in breast.

Lymph nodes. Small, bean-shaped organs located along the lymphatic system. Nodes filter bacteria or cancer cells that may travel through the lymphatic system. Also called lymph glands.

Lymphoma. Primary cancer of the lymph nodes.

Magnetic resonance imaging (MRI). Radiologic study that utilizes a magnet to generate cross-sectional images of the body. Gives excellent detail about soft-tissue densities. Used to detect bone cancer and other conditions, and to evaluate breast implants.

Malignant. Cancerous.

Mammogram. An X ray of the breast.

Margins of resection. Cut edges of the specimen taken out during biopsy; edges of the excision (excised tissue). These are checked for the presence of tumor cells; if no cancer has reached the edge of the tissue, margins are called clean.

Mass. A term used to describe a lesion, tumor, lump, nodule.

Mastectomy. Surgery to remove the breast.

Megace. Brand name for megestrol, a drug used as hormone therapy to control breast cancer. Sometimes used when tamoxifen is ineffective.

Metastasis. The spread of cancer from one part of the body to another.

Metastatic disease. Cancer that has spread from its original site to other parts of the body. Most commonly to bone, lung, liver, brain, lymph nodes.

Metastatic lesion. A cancerous lesion or tumor at another site that has the same cancer cells as the original tumor.

Methotrexate. A cytotoxic drug used to treat breast cancer. The "M" in CMF (see entry).

Microinvasive cancer. Cancer that has less than 5 or 10 percent showing invasion. The rest is noninvasive.

Micrometastasis. Less than 2 millimeters of metastasis in a lymph node.

Microsurgery. Surgical procedure that requires a microscope to perform. Used to suture blood vessels in breast reconstruction.

Modified radical mastectomy. Surgical removal of breast, lymph nodes, nipple/areola complex, pectoralis minor muscle.

Mrad. A unit of measure for radiation; 0.001 rad.

MRI. See *magnetic resonance imaging*.

Multicentric breast cancer. Cancer lesions or cells appearing in more than one quadrant of the breast.

Multifocal breast cancer. Cancer lesions or cells appearing several places within the same quadrant of the breast.

Necrosis. The presence of dead cells.

Needle-guided biopsy. Biopsy of small nonpalpable lesions in which surgeon is guided to the site of the lesions by a needle placed in the breast on the basis of mammogram images.

Negative nodes. Lymph nodes showing no signs of cancer.

Neoadjuvant chemotherapy. Chemotherapy given before surgery to shrink the tumor and facilitate surgery, and also to control metastasis. Sometimes called induction therapy.

Neoplasia. Proliferation of cells whose growth exceeds and is uncoordinated with other cells.

Nolvadex. See *tamoxifen*.

Noninvasive cancer. In situ cancer; a cancer that does not spread to neighboring tissue.

Oncogene. A gene that may promote cancer.

Oncologist. A doctor who specializes in treating cancer (medical oncologist, surgical oncologist, radiation oncologist, etc.).

Osteoporosis. Degenerative bone disease, a demineralization or loss of bone mass, that sometimes develops after menopause when the body no longer produces estrogen.

Paget's disease. A rare form of breast cancer starting in the nipple, usually in situ.

Palliative. Relieves symptoms such as pain. Does not cure.

Palpate. To touch. A simple technique in which the pads of the fingers press lightly on the surface of the body to feel the organs or tissues underneath.

Papilloma. A benign growth in the breast ducts which is very vascular and is the number one cause of blood discharge from the nipple.

Pathologic diagnosis. A histologic diagnosis; a report on the state of the microscopic particles of the tumor.

Pathologist. A doctor who identifies diseases by studying cells and tissues under a microscope.

Pectoralis major. The large muscle behind the breast that covers the chest.

Pectoralis minor. The smaller muscle that is found behind the breast and behind the pectoralis major muscle.

Pedicle flap. A piece of muscle and skin taken from another part of the body to reconstruct the breast. The flap remains attached to its original site by one end and is repositioned onto the chest wall.

Permanent section. The tissue removed during biopsy that is preserved for thorough study. Also, name given the final report after full pathologic evaluation.

Ploidy. DNA measurement in tumor cells.

Port. A small device that is implanted under the skin with a catheter which enters the vessels of the chest and into which medications can be infused. Infusaport.

Positive lymph nodes. Lymph nodes that contain cancer cells.

Premalignant. Indicating a significant potential for cancer.

Primary tumor. The original site of the cancer.

Progesterone. A female hormone.

Progesterone receptor. A protein on the tumor cell surface that binds with progesterone.

Prognostic indicators. All elements of the disease used to determine prognosis (the prospect of recovery) and treatment, such as size and location of the tumor and behavior of the cells involved, number of positive nodes, patient's age, S phase, ploidy, hormone receptor status, etc.

Prophylactic mastectomy. Surgical removal of a breast in order to prevent breast cancer.

Prophylactic tamoxifen. The use of tamoxifen to prevent breast cancer.

Prosthesis. An artificial breast form worn under clothing.

Quadrant. One of the four areas of the breast, described as upper outer, upper inner, lower outer, and lower inner quadrants. Central location means behind the nipple.

Quadrantectomy. A partial mastectomy that removes one quarter of the breast, a treatment not used much anymore.

Rad. A unit of measurement for radiation absorbed by the body. A chest X ray or mammogram delivers a fraction of a rad.

Radiation oncologist. A physician who specializes in radiation treatment for cancer.

Radiation therapy. Treatment with high-energy rays from X rays or other sources to kill or slow cancer cells. Also will reduce pain from cancer spread to bone by killing tumor at this site.

Radical mastectomy. Surgical removal of breast, chest muscles, and lymph nodes.

Radiologist. A physician who specializes in diagnoses with X ray.

Reconstruction. Rebuilding a breast with an implant or human tissue to replace a surgically removed breast.

Rectus abdominus. Abdomen muscle used in TRAM flap reconstruction.

Re-excision. Surgical excision over an area previously biopsied.

RTX. Medical shorthand for radiation treatment. Also written XRT.

RU-486. A drug used for breast cancer; it works against hormones, more specifically, progesterone. Similar to tamoxifen.

Saline implant. A silicone bag filled with salt water (or saline) used in breast reconstruction.

Sarcoma. A rare, often large and aggressive malignancy that grows in the connective tissue of the breast.

Scatter. Radiation that bounces off cells to other parts of the body.

Seroma. A collection of fluid in the axilla or skin after mastectomy. Treated by aspiration, that is, draining with needle and syringe.

Silicone implant. A silicone bag filled with silicone, once used in breast reconstruction; currently under investigation for toxicity.

Simple mastectomy. Removal of the breast without removing any muscles or lymph nodes.

Specimen X ray. X ray taken of the tissue removed at the time of biopsy.

Staging. The process of learning whether cancer has spread from its original site to another part of the body. Clinical stage is based upon history and physical examination. Pathologic stage is based upon findings under the microscope.

Sternum. Breastbone.

Superior vena cava. Blood vessel in the central portion of the chest which delivers blood from the rest of the body to the heart.

Supraclavicular. Term used to describe lymph nodes (or any condition) in the area above the collarbone.

Synchronous. Appearing at the same time. A term used to refer to bilateral breast cancer. *Metachronous* is at different times, maybe a year apart.

Systemic therapy. Treatment that goes through the system, usually via the blood, and reaches and affects cells all over the body.

Tamoxifen. An antiestrogen that is used as adjuvant chemotherapy to form a barrier between estrogen and cancer cells. Used to prevent recurrence of breast cancer and may help prevent the development of breast cancer. Sold under the brand name Nolvadex.   .

Taxol. A drug made from yew tree bark for cytotoxic chemotherapy.

Tissue expander. A breast implant that is gradually inflated with saline over a period of months to force the skin to expand to a certain size. Then usually replaced with a permanent implant.

TRAM flap. The transverse rectus abdominus muscle, used to reconstruct the breast. It is severed at the bottom of the abdomen, pulled up through the ribs, and formed into a breast.

Transillumination. An infrared light used to see into the breasts.

Tumor. A mass of tissue, lesion, lump, nodule.

Tx. Medical shorthand for "treatment." Also written Rx.

Ultrasound. A diagnostic test that bounces sound waves off tissues and converts the echoes into pictures.

Unilateral. One-sided.

Wedge resection. A form of partial mastectomy in which a pie-shaped piece of the breast is removed; rarely used, given current standard for lumpectomy and axillary dissection.

Xeroradiography. An inferior type of mammography that records the picture of the breast on paper rather than on film.

X ray. Low-energy radiation; used in low doses to diagnose disease; also used at high energy levels in high doses to treat cancer.

Zofran. A medication to alleviate nausea caused by cytotoxic chemotherapy.

INDEX

lymphedema (cont.)
    arm's baseline measurement and, 165,
        176–177
    axillary dissection and, 59, 64
    diet and, 171
    exercises for, 165–171, 176
    infection and, 172–173
    massage and, 173–174, 177
    occurrence of, 164–165
    organizations for information on, 175
    pneumatic pump for, 174
    questions to ask about, 176–177
    salt and, 172
    self-screening and, 165
    support sleeve for, 172, 177
    trauma and, 173
    weather and, 171–172
lymph nodes, 9, 164
    axillary dissection of, see axillary
        dissection
    biopsy and status of, 31
    cervical, 54
    chemotherapy and, 55, 105, 106
    diagnosis and, 32
    follow-up care and, 151
    function of, 54
    infraclavicular, 54
    negative, 55
    positive, 35, 55, 92
    as prognostic indicator, 53–54
    radiation therapy and, 87, 97
    swollen, 12, 54–55
    types of, 54
lymphoma, 13, 97

magnetic resonance imaging (MRI), 20
major pectoralis muscle, 53
male breast cancer, 14
mammary lymph nodes, 54
mammograms:
    additional views in, 17
    bilateral, 98, 139
    corporate sponsors of, 191
    cost of, 18–19, 22
    detection of lump and, 4, 5
    discovery and, 4, 5
    ductal carcinoma in situ (DCIS) and,
        10, 49
    facilities for, 16, 18
    film screen method of, 15–16, 22
    follow-up care and, 149, 150, 151, 155
    free, 191
    implants and, 17
    interpretation of, 17–18, 22–23
    low cost, 191

lumpectomy and, 11–12
    medical insurance and, 18
    ownership of, 19, 22
    premalignant conditions and, 8
    proper compression and, 17
    questions to ask about, 21–23
    radiation dose in, 16
    role of, 15
    screening and, 138, 162
    standard workup of, 16–17
    technicians and, 21
margins of resection, 30, 35, 106
marijuana, 112
massage:
    implants and, 70
    manual lymph drainage (MLD) system
        of, 173–174, 177
    physical therapy and, 174
mastectomy, 6, 13, 36, 41, 129
    bilateral, 12
    bras and, 82
    breast self-exam after, 80
    breast size and, 52
    elderly women and, 48
    hospitalization and, 58
    implants after, 69–71
    incisions for, 57, 62
    informed consent laws and, 48–49
    lumpectomy vs., 49–50, 51
    lymph node removal and, 53–54
    modified radical, 52, 53
    in Northeast vs. South and Midwest, 47
    Paget's disease and, 11
    partial, 51
    pectoralis muscles and, 57
    during pregnancy, 137–138
    prophylactic, 66–67, 81
    radiation therapy and, 87–88
    reconstruction after, 69–71
    reconstruction with, 42, 58, 67, 68, 84
    recovery from, 59–60
    recurrence and, 163
    simple, 9
    surviving breast and, 67
    types of, 52–53
mastitis, 11
MDR-1 (multiple drug resistance) gene, 31
Medicaid, 81, 100
Medic Alert, 72
medical insurance:
    Americans with Disabilities Act and,
        194–195
    biofeedback and, 145
    chemotherapy and, 125
    employment and, 194–195

About the Authors

Lydia Komarnicky, M.D., and **Anne Rosenberg, M.D.,** are physicians who have devoted themselves to the treatment of breast cancer. Both are young women and mothers who have become leaders in the healthcare community and advocates of the breast cancer cause. They are advisers to the Linda Creed Breast Cancer Foundation and have appeared on radio and television programs to talk about breast cancer.

Dr. Komarnicky is a radiation oncologist at Lankenau Hospital in Philadelphia and an assistant professor at Thomas Jefferson Medical College. She is part of a group studying ways to help disadvantaged women and belongs to a research task force of the National Alliance of Breast Cancer Organizations (NABCO). She sits on various national committees of radiologists and has written extensively on breast cancer.

Dr. Rosenberg is the preeminent breast surgeon of the Philadelphia area. That's the only type of surgery she does — or has ever done since completing her medical training. She sits on several professional committees for the study and treatment of breast cancer and teaches breast surgery at Jefferson Medical College. She practices at Thomas Jefferson University Hospital in Philadelphia and Our Lady of Lourdes Hospital in Camden, New Jersey. Dr. Rosenberg has been honored by several national boards of surgeons.

Marian Betancourt has been a professional writer and editor for more than twenty years. Her work has appeared in national magazines and newspapers. Since 1990 she has written extensively about medical issues as an editor and writer at Thomas Jefferson University. She has had a special interest in breast cancer since her own bout with it in 1992. She is a member of the American Society of Journalists and Authors and the Authors Guild. She is a native New Yorker and lives in Brooklyn.